AGING
HEALTHY
AND
YOUNGER LOOK

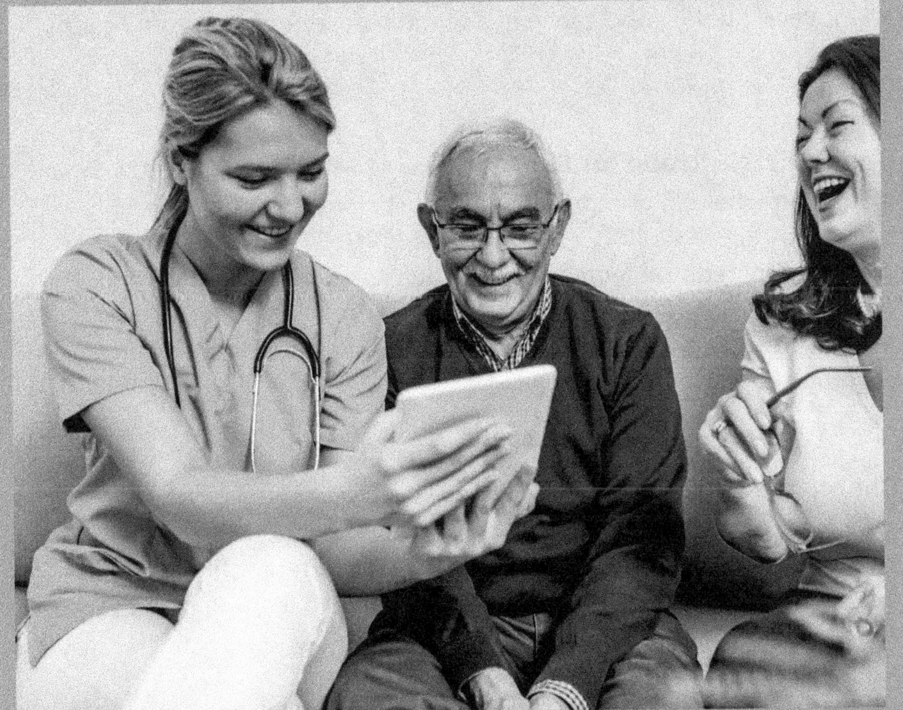

*Strategies for Maintaining Health and Fitness
as You Age*

SERENA .M. MERVIL

Table of content

Introduction

Brief overview of the importance of maintaining health and fitness as individuals age
Acknowledgment of the common challenges associated with aging
Introduction to the holistic approach to healthy aging

Chapter 1: Understanding the Aging Process
- Overview of the physiological changes that occur with aging
- Discussion on the impact of aging on metabolism, muscle mass, and bone density
- Emphasis on the importance of adapting lifestyle to promote healthy aging

Chapter 2: Nutrition for Longevity
- Exploring the role of nutrition in supporting overall health as individuals age
- Nutritional requirements for aging adults, including vitamins and minerals
- Dietary recommendations to promote energy, bone health, and cognitive function

Chapter 3: Exercise for Aging Well
- Benefits of regular exercise for aging individuals
- Tailoring exercise routines to accommodate different fitness levels
- Incorporating strength training, flexibility exercises, and cardiovascular activities

Chapter 4: Mental Fitness and Cognitive Health
- Discussing the connection between mental and physical health
- Strategies for maintaining cognitive function and preventing age-related cognitive decline
- Activities and exercises to stimulate the brain and promote mental well-being

Chapter 5: Sleep and Recovery
- Importance of quality sleep for overall health
- Tips for improving sleep hygiene
- Exploring the role of sleep in muscle recovery and immune function

Chapter 6: Managing Stress for Healthy Aging
- Understanding the impact of stress on aging
- Stress-reduction techniques, including mindfulness and relaxation exercises
- Creating a balanced and stress-resilient lifestyle

Chapter 7: Social Connections and Emotional Well-being
- Exploring the role of social relationships in healthy aging
- Strategies for maintaining and fostering social connections
- Addressing emotional well-being and mental health in the aging population

Chapter 8: Preventive Health Measures
- Overview of preventive health screenings and vaccinations for older adults
- The importance of regular health check-ups and early detection of age-related health issues
- Tips for proactive health management and disease prevention

Chapter 9: Adapting to Lifestyle Changes
- Discussing the importance of adapting to changing circumstances and abilities
- Strategies for maintaining independence and quality of life
Resources and support systems for aging individuals and their families

Conclusion
Summarizing key strategies for healthy aging discussed in the
book
Encouraging a proactive and positive approach to aging
Reinforcing the importance of a holistic lifestyle for maintaining
health and fitness in the later years

Appendix
Additional resources, references, and recommended reading for
further
exploration

"Healthy Aging: Strategies for Maintaining Health and Fitness as You Age," an inspirational journey into the art of aging with grace, resilience, and energy, is now available. We shall examine each of the three pillars that support a comprehensive and long-lasting approach to healthy aging. These three pillars serve as the basis for this guide.

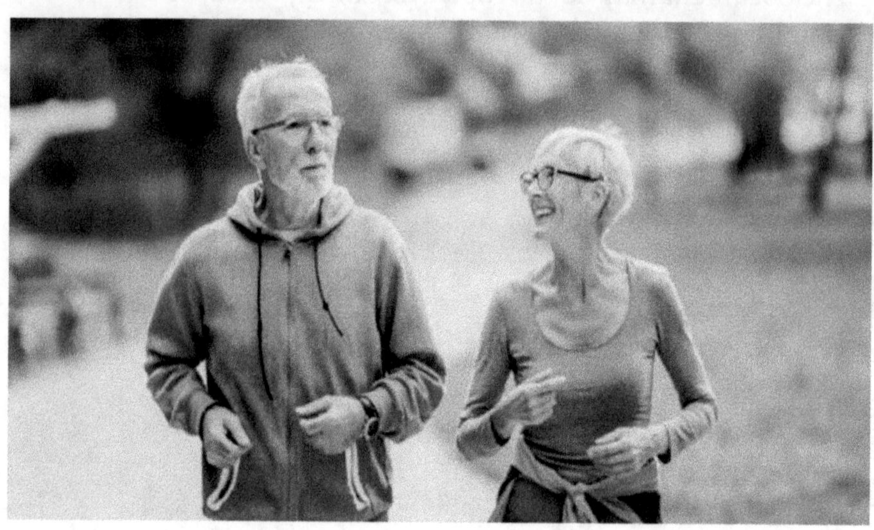

The Importance of Maintaining Health and Fitness

Keeping ourselves physically and mentally fit is becoming more and more important as time progresses and we navigate the complex fabric of life. This book begins with an analysis of the critical significance of adopting a way of life that promotes mental and physical health at an early age.

Together, we will discover the keys to releasing our bodies' and minds' greatest potential and building a foundation that will enable us to enjoy life to the fullest at every turn.

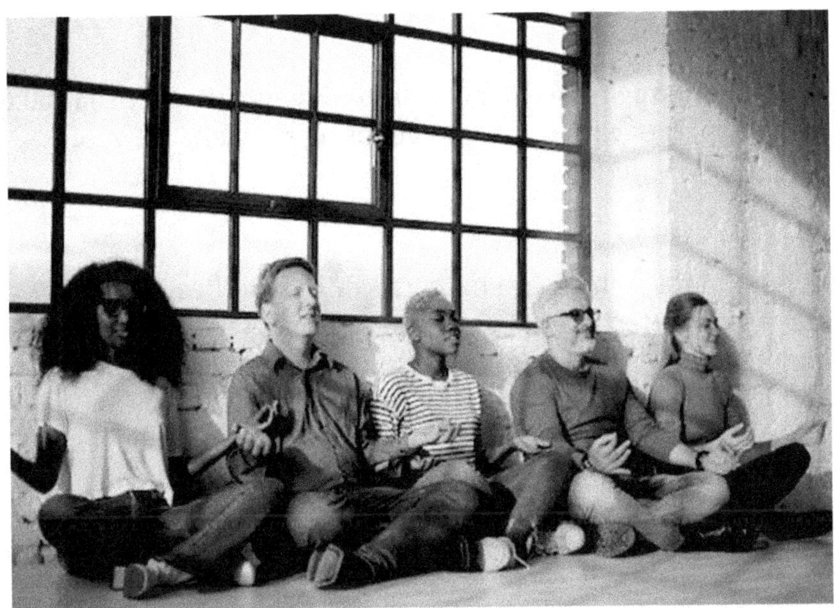

Recognizing the Typical Obstacles Associated with Getting Older

Although it is a common experience, growing older comes with a unique set of problems. This book offers a sympathetic recognition of these difficulties, regardless of how they appear as modifications to bone density, muscle mass, or metabolism.
By identifying and comprehending these typical obstacles, we open the door to customized plans and well-informed decisions that can improve the quality of our aging process.

Overview of the Holistic Approach to Age-Responsible Living
The process of aging is multifaceted and involves aspects of mental, emotional, and physical health. The idea of holistic, healthy aging—a complete strategy that recognizes the interdependence of these aspects—is presented in this handbook.

We want to help you live a balanced, harmonious existence that takes care of every part of who you are by adopting a holistic viewpoint.

Let's now explore each of the chapters, which have been painstakingly written to offer advice, techniques, and doable recommendations for attaining and preserving fitness and health as you age. This guide is your partner in the quest for a happy and full life as you age, from comprehending the physiological changes in Chapter 1 to adopting preventative health measures in Chapter

Chapter One: Understanding the Aging Process

Growing older is a normal and unavoidable stage in life's vast tapestry, a journey symbolized by time's exquisite waltz across the canvas of our existence.

As we embark on this journey of healthy aging, it is critical to first grasp the complexities of the aging process, including the subtle yet profound changes that occur within our bodies and minds.

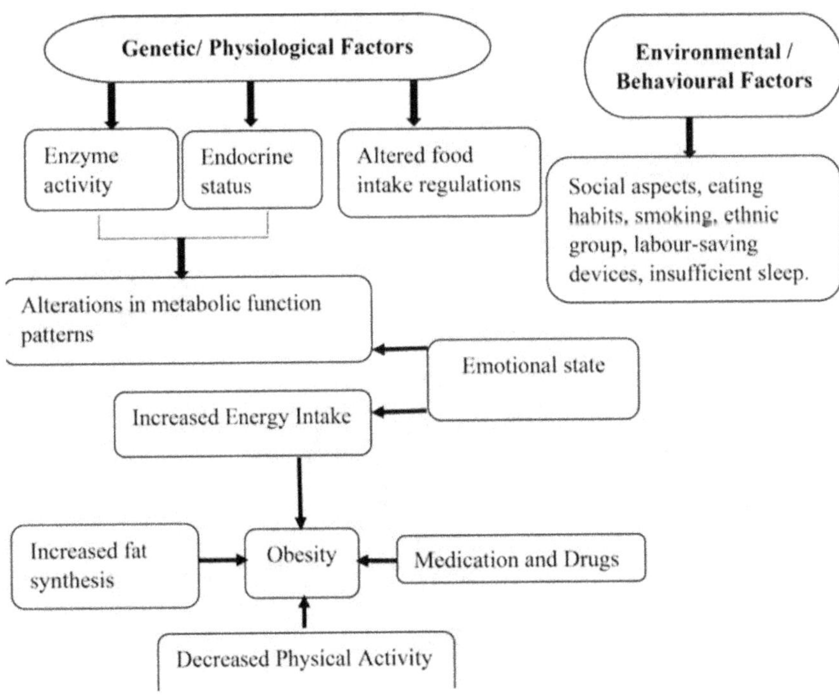

1. Overview of Physiological Changes Associated with Aging

Aging, at its core, is a symphony of physiological changes. Our bodies undergo change, gently

managing the passage of time. Cellular processes decelerate, and organs may exhibit modest changes in function.

Understanding these shifts provides the compass that guides us toward specific methods for preserving optimal health over time.

This chapter acts as a guidebook, providing light on the subtle changes that create the aging process and ultimately equipping you to manage this trip with wisdom and grace.

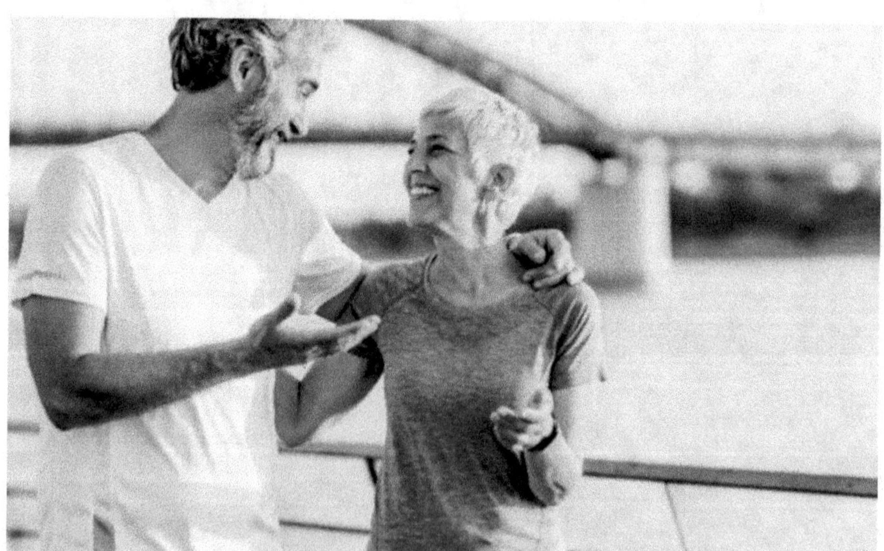

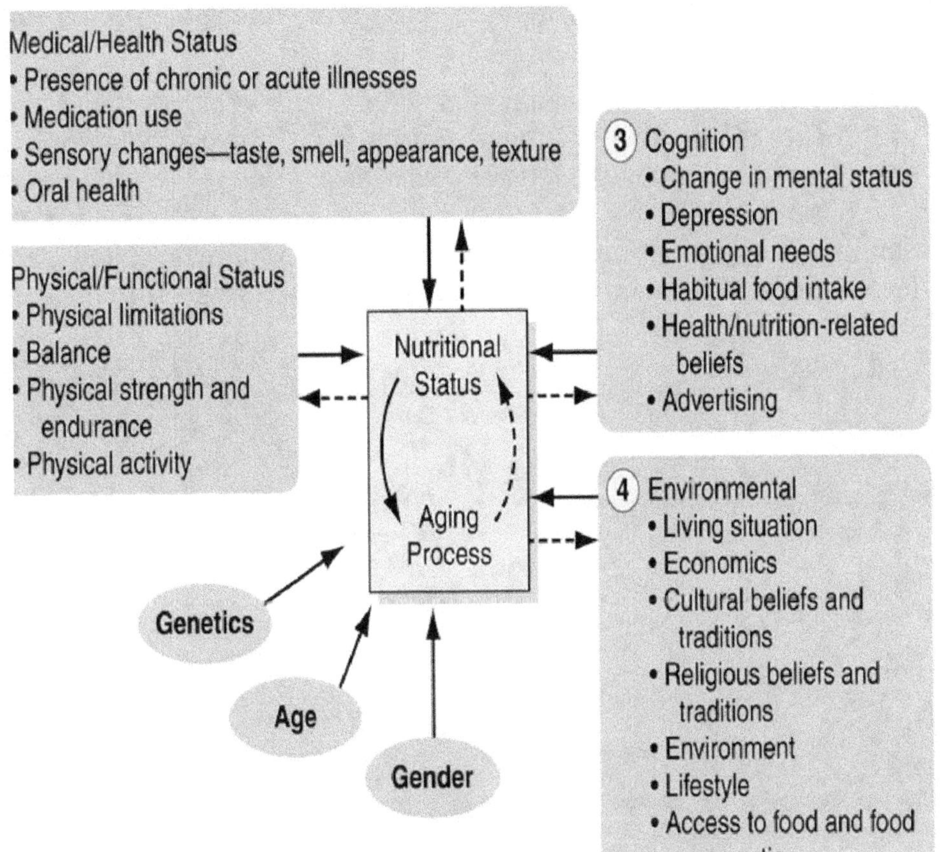

Medical/Health Status
• Presence of chronic or acute illnesses
• Medication use
• Sensory changes—taste, smell, appearance, texture
• Oral health
Physical/Functional Status
• Physical limitations
• Balance
• Physical strength and endurance
• Physical activity
Genetics
Age
Gender
Nutritional Status
Aging Process
3 Cognition
• Change in mental status
• Depression
• Emotional needs
• Habitual food intake
• Health/nutrition-related beliefs
• Advertising
4 Environmental
• Living situation
• Economics
• Cultural beliefs and traditions
• Religious beliefs and traditions
• Environment
• Lifestyle
• Access to food and food

2. The effect of aging on metabolism, muscle mass, and bone density.

One of the most visible aspects of aging is its effect on critical aspects of our physique, such as metabolism,

muscle mass, and bone density. Metabolism, once a fervent flame, may flicker more slowly with age. Muscle mass, the custodian of our strength and mobility, deteriorates over time.

Simultaneously, the framework of our skeletal system, our bones, undergoes alterations that might have an impact on posture and structural integrity.

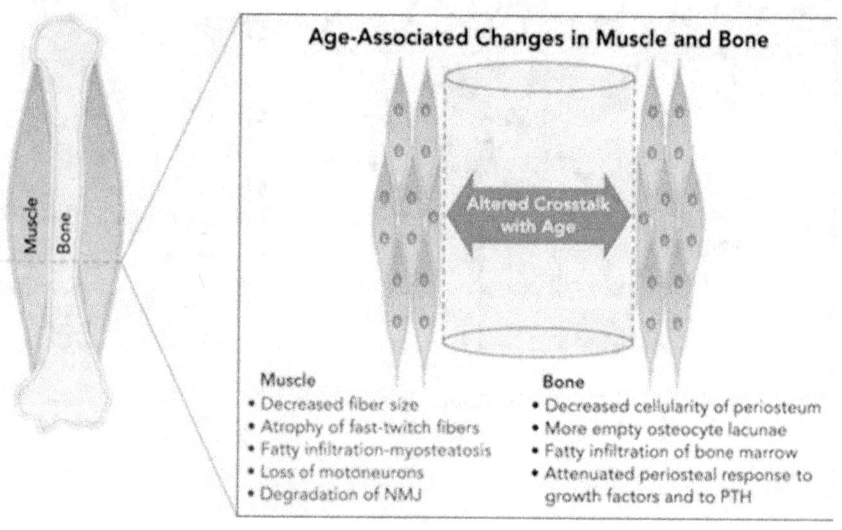

In this chapter, we will take a thoughtful look at these changes, recognizing their implications and, more importantly, determining how we might proactively mitigate their effects through conscious lifestyle choices.

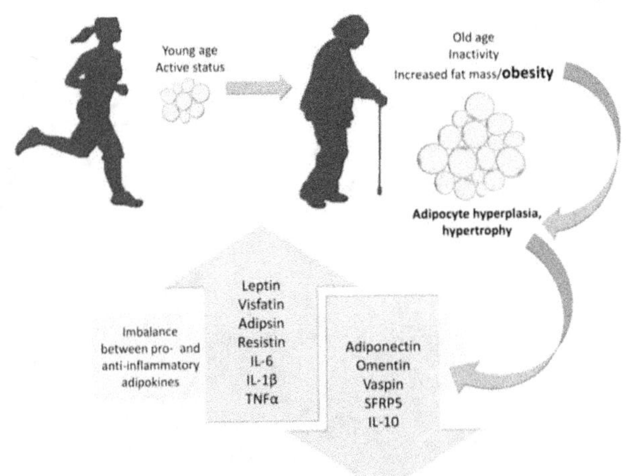

3. Emphasis on the Importance of Lifestyle Changes to Promote Healthy Aging.

As we learn more about the physiological subtleties of aging, we discover an important truth: our lifestyle choices have a significant impact on the trajectory of our health.

The art of graceful aging is based on our ability to adapt and build a lifestyle that matches our bodies' changing requirements.

This chapter emphasizes the significance of accepting change and making informed decisions regarding nutrition, exercise, and overall health. By adopting

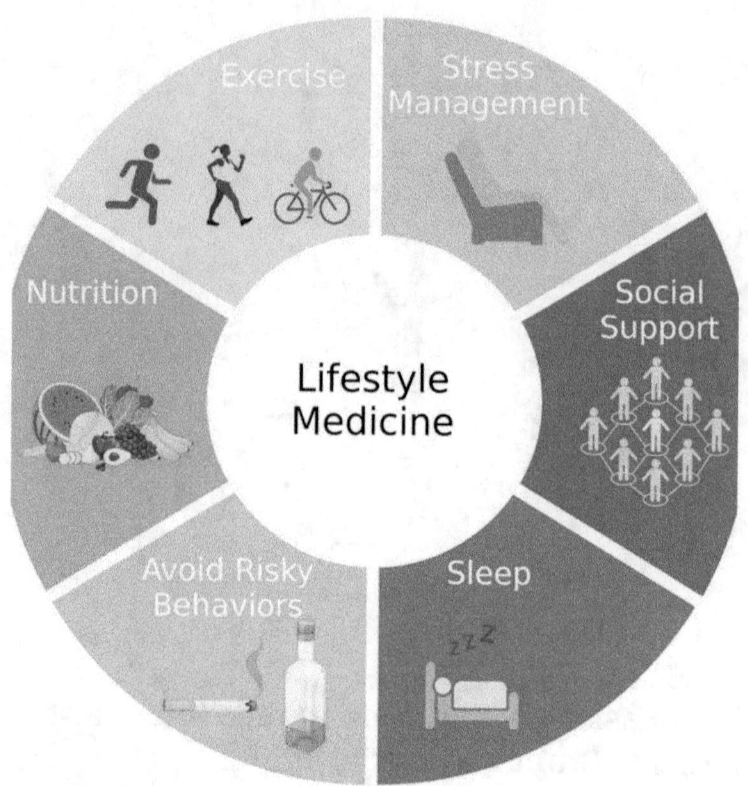

practices that encourage resilience and vitality, we can age with strength and purpose.

Understanding the aging process is essential for ensuring healthy living. Aging is a normal and unavoidable part of life, and understanding its physiological and psychological elements can help people make educated decisions about their health and well-being. Here are some important aspects of understanding the aging process and its implications for healthy living:

Physiological Changes:

Individuals' bodies undergo a variety of physiological changes as they age. These can include changes in muscle mass, bone density, metabolism, and organ function.

Understanding these changes enables people to modify their lifestyle to meet the special needs associated with aging.

Metabolism and nutrition:

Metabolic rates frequently decline with age, limiting the body's ability to digest and utilize nutrients properly.

Being aware of these changes allows you to make more informed food choices and ensures you get enough nourishment to stay healthy.

Muscle mass and bone density

As we get older, our muscles and bones naturally lose some of their bulk and density, making us more prone to fractures and limiting our mobility.

Regular exercise, particularly strength training, can reduce these impacts and promote good aging.

Empowerment and proactivity:

Knowing more about aging gives people more control over their health.

Proactive steps, such as living a healthy lifestyle, obtaining preventative treatment, and remaining knowledgeable about health-related decisions, help to improve overall health.

Quality of life:

Finally, understanding the aging process leads to a higher quality of life in later years.

Individuals can live full and healthy lives if they embrace the changes and challenges of aging with knowledge and a good attitude.

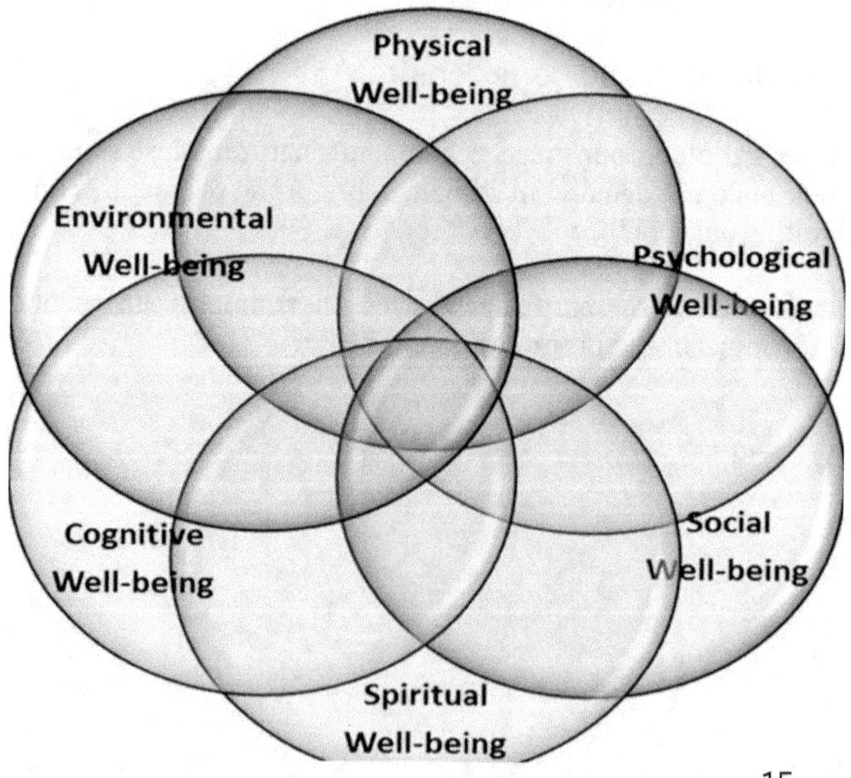

To summarize, understanding the aging process is essential for maintaining a healthy lifestyle. It enables people to traverse the aging process with awareness, adaptation, and a dedication to preserving general well-being at all phases of life.

In the following pages, we will go further into actionable tactics and empowering insights, building on this foundation of knowledge. Remember that each passing year provides an opportunity to redefine and improve our approach to health. Let us embrace the wisdom that comes with age and chart a course for healthy aging—one that appreciates the beauty of every stage

Chapter 2: Eating to Live Longer

Healthy aging is like a fine tapestry, and diet is like the master brushstroke that weaves its way through the fabric of our health. It becomes more and more clear as time goes on how important it is to eat a healthy diet.

Come with us on a journey through Chapter 2, where we'll talk about the important role that nutrition plays in extending life, the special nutritional needs of older adults, and practical ways to improve your energy, bone health, and brain function.

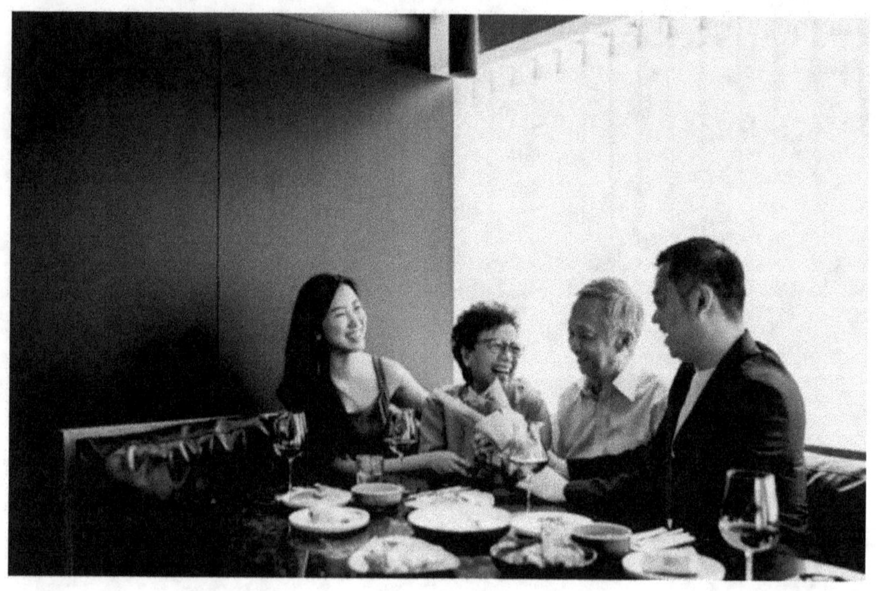

1. Looking into how nutrition can help people stay healthy as they age

Nutrition is important for our health in many ways, including our mental and physical health. As we get older, it becomes more and more important to intentionally feed our bodies. This chapter wants you to learn more about the complicated link between what you eat and your health as a whole. From supporting the immune system to maintaining organ function, nutrition works as a catalyst for a thriving and resilient body.

We delve into the profound effect of food choices on the aging process, empowering you to make informed decisions that resonate with the essence of healthy aging.

2. Nutritional Requirements for Aging Adults, Including Vitamins and Minerals

Aging introduces subtle shifts in the body's nutritional needs, necessitating a keen knowledge of the vitamins and minerals essential for vitality.

This section offers a comprehensive guide to the unique nutritional requirements of aging adults. Delving into the intricacies of micronutrients, we study how vitamins and minerals contribute to bone health, cognitive function, and overall longevity. Armed with this information, you can tailor your dietary choices to meet the unique demands of the aging body, fortifying your health from within.

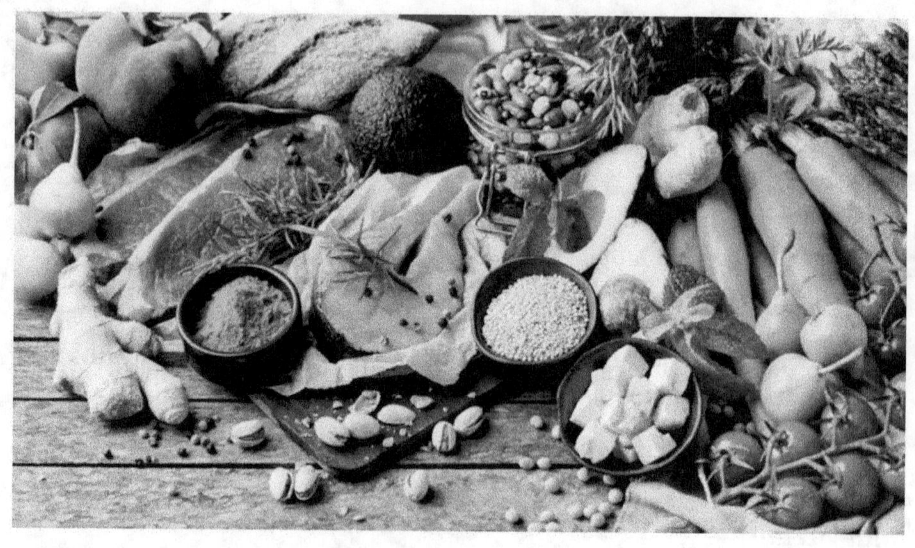

3. Dietary Recommendations to Promote Energy, Bone Health, and Cognitive Function

The decisions we make at the dining table reverberate through the years, affecting our energy levels, bone density, and cognitive prowess.

This chapter extends a hand of guidance, giving practical and achievable dietary advice to optimize your nutritional intake. From foods that fuel sustained energy to those that support robust bone health and cognitive function, we uncover the secrets to a well-rounded and longevity-focused diet.

Discover how simple modifications to your daily meals can become powerful tools in your quest for sustained health and energy.

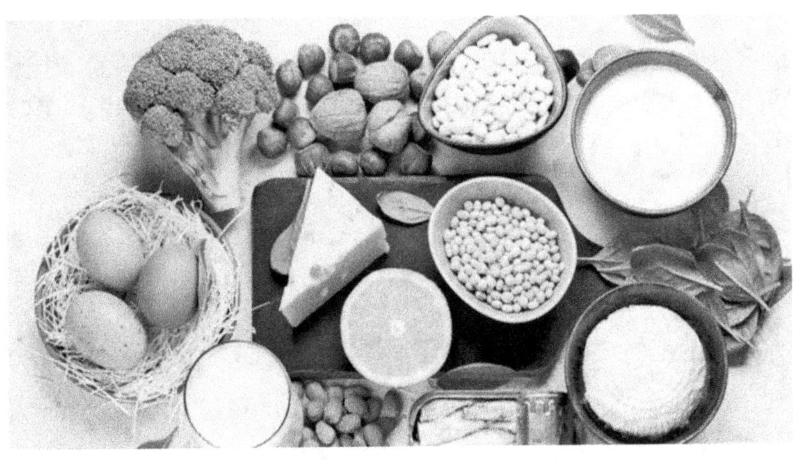

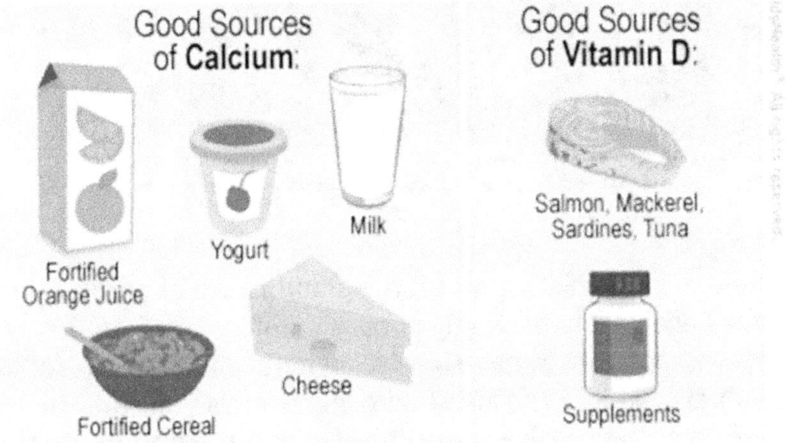

As we start on this nutritional odyssey, remember that each bite is a step toward a future of resilient well-being. Join us in unlocking the potential of nutrition for longevity, and let the journey toward good aging be one adorned with wholesome, nourishing choices.

Chapter 3: Exercise for Aging Well

In the harmonious symphony of healthy aging, the rhythm of exercise echoes as a cornerstone melody, weaving vitality into the very fabric of our existence.

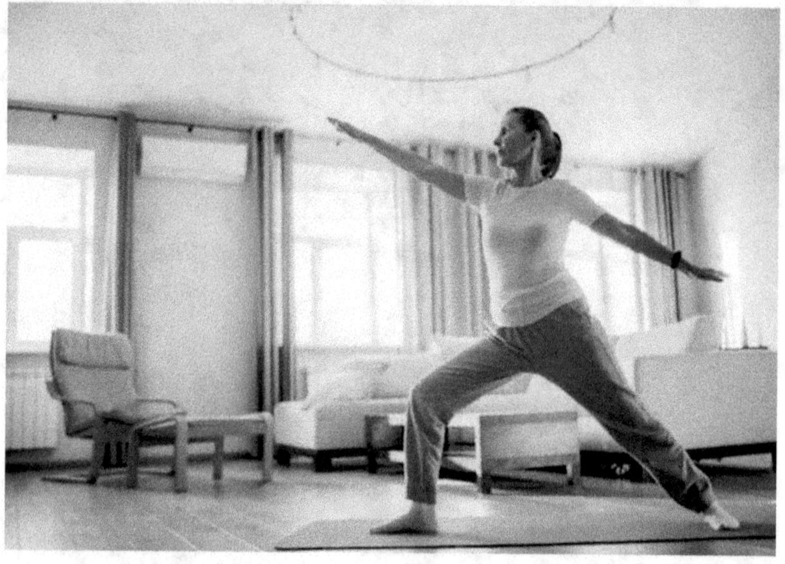

As the years gracefully unfold, the significance of regular physical activity becomes increasingly apparent. Join us in Chapter 3, where we illuminate the transformative benefits of exercise for aging individuals, explore the art of tailoring exercise routines to diverse fitness levels, and delve into the seamless integration of strength training, flexibility exercises, and cardiovascular activities.

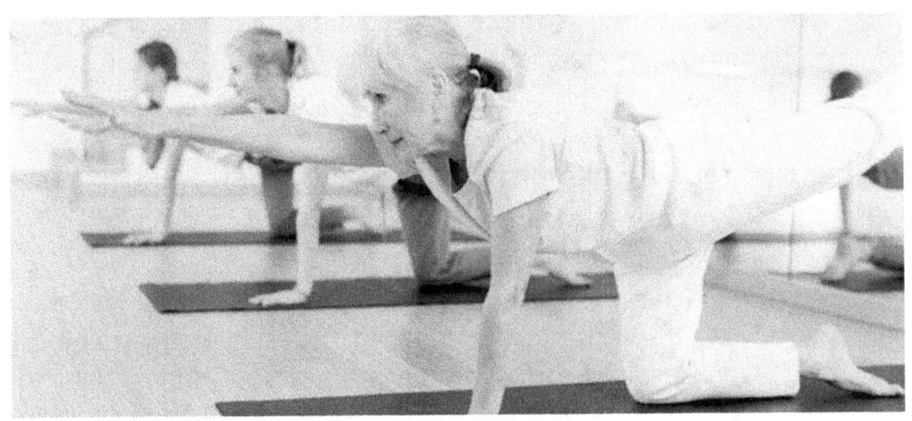

1. Benefits of Regular Exercise for Aging Individuals

The power of movement transcends the boundaries of age, infusing life with vigor and resilience. This section unravels the profound benefits of regular exercise, specifically tailored for aging individuals. From enhanced cardiovascular health to improved mood and cognitive function, the positive impact of physical activity on overall well-being is both diverse and transformative. We explore how a commitment to movement can be a steadfast companion in your journey toward healthy aging, promoting not only physical strength but also mental and emotional vitality.

2. Tailoring Exercise Routines to Accommodate Different Fitness Levels

Recognizing the unique tapestry of fitness levels within the aging population, this chapter guides you in tailoring exercise routines to suit individual needs and capabilities. Whether you are a seasoned fitness enthusiast or just beginning your journey, the importance lies in creating a sustainable and personalized exercise plan. We delve into the art of crafting routines that are accessible, enjoyable, and adaptable, ensuring that everyone, regardless of their starting point, can embrace the benefits of physical activity.

3. Incorporating Strength Training, Flexibility Exercises, and Cardiovascular Activities

A holistic approach to exercise for aging well involves the integration of three fundamental elements: strength training, flexibility exercises, and cardiovascular activities. Strength training preserves and builds muscle mass, fostering resilience and mobility. Flexibility exercises enhance joint mobility and reduce the risk of injuries. Cardiovascular activities elevate heart health, improve circulation, and contribute to overall stamina. This chapter serves as a guide to seamlessly incorporating these elements into your exercise routine, creating a balanced regimen that caters to the multifaceted needs of aging bodies.

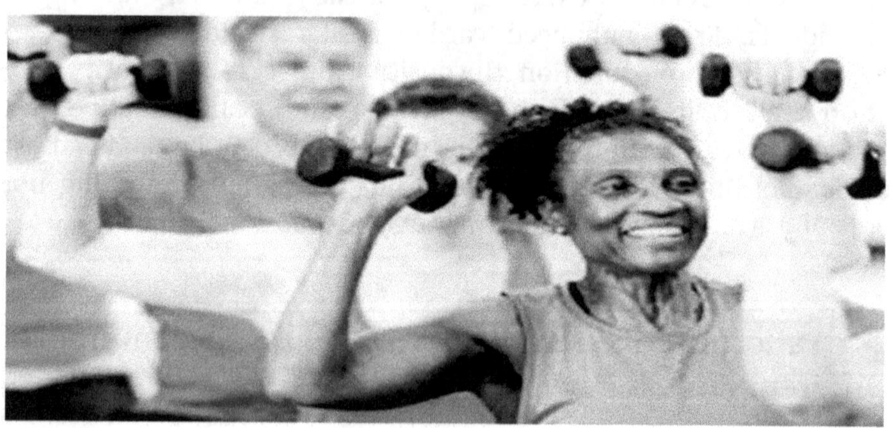

Embark with us on this movement journey, where

each step becomes a celebration of strength, flexibility, and endurance. Through intentional and tailored exercise, we strive to unlock the gates to a future where the body ages well, fortified by the transformative benefits of physical activity. Let the symphony of movement guide you toward a life of vibrancy and resilience.

Some Crucial Aspects of Exercise and Healthy Aging

Maintaining physical health:
Muscular Strength: Regular exercise, particularly resistance or strength training, helps to preserve muscular mass, which naturally declines with age.

Bone Density: Weight-bearing and resistance activities improve bone health, lowering the risk of osteoporosis.

Joint Flexibility: Stretching and flexibility exercises improve joint mobility, lower the risk of injury, and increase overall agility.

Cardiovascular Health

Heart Health: Walking, swimming, and cycling are examples of aerobic exercises that enhance cardiovascular health by lowering the risk of heart disease and fostering effective blood circulation.

Weight Management: Regular physical activity helps with weight management, which is important for overall health and the prevention of diseases such as diabetes.

Cognitive Function:

Brain Health: Exercise has been linked to cognitive benefits such as better memory, attention, and general brain function. It may help lower the risk of cognitive deterioration due to aging.

Emotional Wellbeing:
Stress Reduction: Physical activity causes the release of endorphins, which promote happiness and reduce stress.

Mood Enhancement: Regular exercise can help to decrease feelings of anxiety and despair, hence improving emotional health.

Group Activities: Participating in group workouts, classes, or sports can help you make social

connections and reduce feelings of isolation and loneliness.
Community Involvement: Participating in physical activities in your community allows you to connect with others and gain support.

Adaptability and longevity:
Functional independence is promoted by the maintenance of physical fitness via exercise, which empowers individuals to effortlessly perform routine tasks.

Increased Lifespan: Research indicates that regular exercise is linked to a longer, healthier life.

Personal Approach:

Consultation with Healthcare Professionals: Before beginning any fitness program, it is critical to consult with a healthcare expert, especially if you have pre-existing medical concerns.

Tailored Exercise Plans: Tailoring exercise regimens to individual tastes, fitness levels, and health problems ensures a long-term and joyful physical activity experience.

Chapter 4: Cognitive Health and Mental Fitness

The mind is the conductor of our well-being, performing a masterful role in the complex dance of healthy aging. In Chapter 4, the interdependence of mental and physical health is explored, methods for protecting cognitive function are revealed, and a variety of exercises and activities designed to activate the brain and promote mental health are presented.

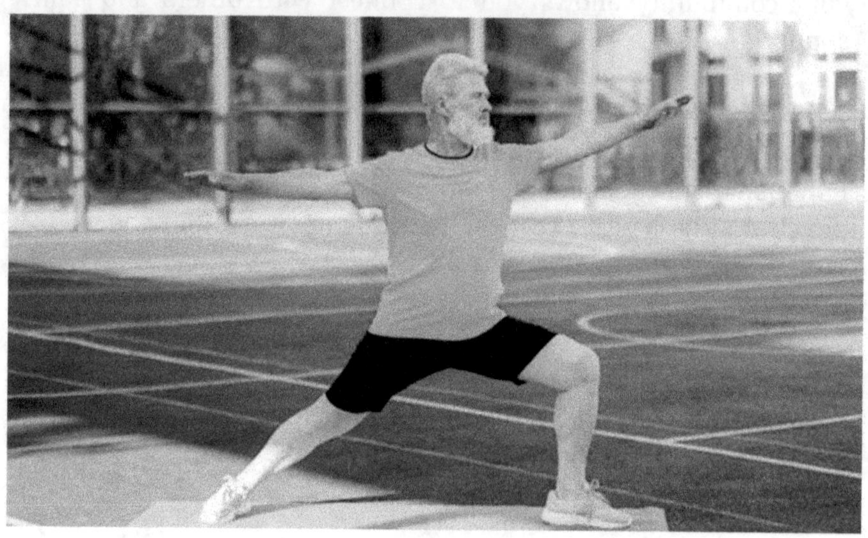

Cognitive health and mental fitness are crucial components of good aging. Here are some techniques for improving cognitive well-being as you age:

Engage in Lifelong Learning:

Continuous Education: Enroll in courses, attend seminars, or pursue hobbies that entail learning new skills. Keeping your mind active and engaged promotes cognitive resilience.

Brain-boosting exercises:

Puzzles and Games: Test your cognitive abilities with puzzles, crosswords, Sudoku, and brain-training apps. These activities activate various parts of the brain and improve mental agility.

Memory Games: Engage in memory-enhancing activities that involve concentration and recall. This can include card games, board games, and digital memory exercises.

Physical Exercise:

Aerobic Activities: Regular physical activity, particularly aerobic activities such as walking, jogging, or swimming, has been associated with better cognitive function and a lower risk of cognitive decline.

Balanced Nutrition:

Brain-Boosting Foods: Eat a range of nutrient-dense foods, including fruits, vegetables, whole grains, and omega-3 fatty acids. These promote brain health and cognitive function.

Adequate Sleep:

Prioritize proper sleep hygiene to ensure that you get enough, high-quality sleep. Sleep is essential for memory consolidation and general cognitive function.

Maintain Social Connections: Participate in social activities to reduce feelings of isolation and loneliness. Meaningful conversations and relationships activate the brain and promote emotional well-being.

Stress Management:

Mindfulness and relaxation techniques: To cope with stress, practice mindfulness meditation, deep breathing techniques, or yoga. Chronic stress might impair cognitive performance; thus, these strategies encourage relaxation.

Stay socially active.

Joining clubs, social groups, or volunteer organizations can help you stay socially engaged. Positive social connections help people feel better and think more clearly.

Cognitive Training Programs:

Brain Training Apps: Discover cognitive training apps that stimulate various brain functions. These apps frequently include activities to increase memory, concentration, and problem-solving abilities.

Regular Health Check-Ups:

Monitoring Overall Health: Regular health check-ups can assist in identifying and treating any medical disorders that may have an impact on cognitive health. Conditions such as hypertension, diabetes, and high cholesterol can impair brain function.

Mind/Body Practices:

Mindfulness and meditation: Practice mindfulness techniques to increase focus, attention, and overall mental health. Meditation can improve brain shape and function.

Social and Emotional Support:

Therapeutic Support: Seek expert help if necessary. Therapists and counselors can help you manage stress, anxiety, and other emotional difficulties.

By adopting these tactics into your daily routine, you can improve cognitive health and mental fitness, fostering a happy and resilient mentality as you age.

1. Talking About the Relationship Between Physical and Mental Health

A key truth that emphasizes the significance of aging gracefully is the symbiotic relationship between mental and physical health. This chapter delves into the complex relationship that exists between a healthy body and a sharp intellect. We explore the complex connections between mental and physical health, including the effects of exercise on cognition and the importance of diet for brain health.

As we go through this conversation, it becomes clear how important it is to take a holistic approach to
health—one that acknowledges the significant impact mental fitness has on the whole picture of good aging.

2. Techniques for Preventing Age-Related Cognitive Decline and Preserving Cognitive Function

As we age, cognitive health becomes an increasingly valuable tool for maintaining a healthy lifestyle.

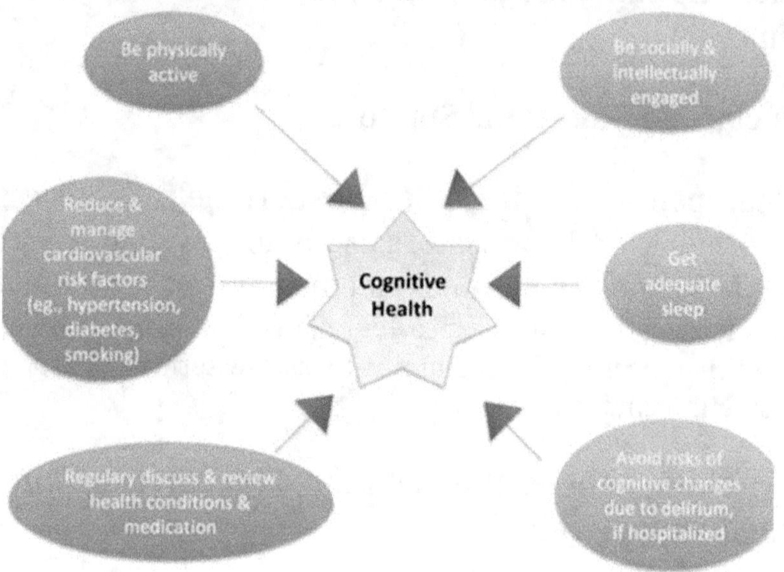

A summary of tactics designed to prevent age-related cognitive decline and preserve cognitive function is provided in this chapter. We look at doable, research-backed strategies that enable you to develop and maintain cognitive vigor, from eating a brain-healthy diet to participating in lifelong learning.

You can actively contribute to creating a future in which mental acuity is still a guiding principle by being aware of the variables that affect cognitive health.

3. Brain-Stimulating Exercises and Activities to Advance Mental Health

The brain is an amazing organ that needs engagement and stimulation to function properly. This section offers a variety of workouts and activities that are meant to stimulate the mind and promote mental health.

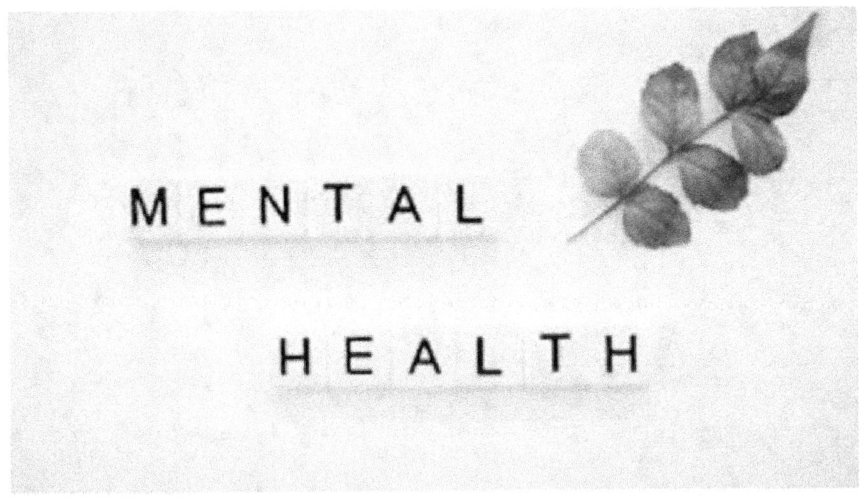

These activities function as a toolset for encouraging a robust and vibrant brain, ranging from puzzles that test cognitive agility to mindfulness exercises that uplift the soul. You may strengthen your mental fortitude and improve your ability to concentrate, remember things, and feel emotionally balanced by practicing the art of stimulation.

Set off on a journey of discovery into mental fitness, where the mind plays an active role in the process of aging in a healthy way, rather than just being a spectator.

Let us accept the wisdom that each exercise and technique reveal as we make our way through the world of cognition. This wisdom will lead us to a future of sustained mental life.

Chapter 5: Sleep and Recovery

The body and mind begin on a remarkable voyage of regeneration during the peaceful hours of the night—an expedition crucial to the tapestry of healthy aging. Chapter 5 deconstructs the relevance of quality sleep, provides helpful advice for improving sleep hygiene, and investigates the critical role of sleep-in muscle recovery and immune function.

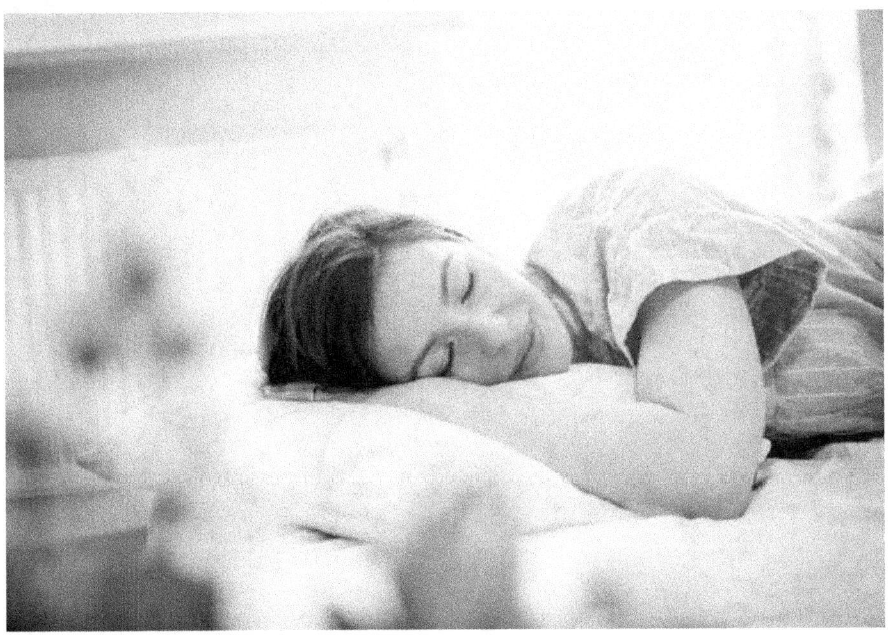

1. The Importance of Good Sleep for Overall Health

Sleep is a cornerstone of holistic well-being, a haven where the body and mind may rejuvenate and heal themselves. This section dives into the critical role of healthy sleep-in overall health, emphasizing its impact on physical, mental, and emotional vigor. From cognitive performance to emotional resilience, the benefits of adequate sleep extend far beyond the nighttime hours, laying the groundwork for a healthy and resilient existence.

2. Sleep Hygiene Improvement Tips

Creating an environment conducive to restful sleep entails practicing good sleep hygiene. This chapter provides a collection of practical recommendations for improving your sleep environment and promoting greater sleep quality. From building a peaceful nighttime routine to establishing a consistent sleep schedule, these ideas enable you to take charge of your sleep health. By adopting these behaviors into your bedtime routine, you set the stage for a comfortable night's sleep, nurturing your body and mind in preparation for the day ahead.

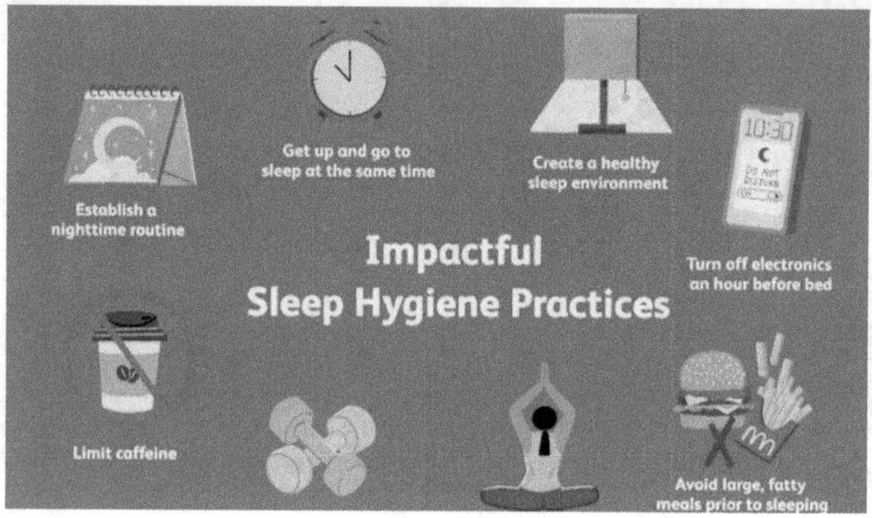

3. Investigating Sleep's Role in Muscle Recovery and Immune Function

As we delve deeper into the realms of sleep, we discover its complex significance in two critical areas of health: muscle recuperation and immunological function. This section explains how sleep contributes to muscle repair and regeneration, which is essential for maintaining strength and resilience. Furthermore, we investigate the substantial impact of sleep on immunological function, shedding light on the relationship between peaceful slumber and the body's ability to protect against sickness. Understanding these connections provides insight into the critical role that quality sleep plays in bolstering your physical well-being.

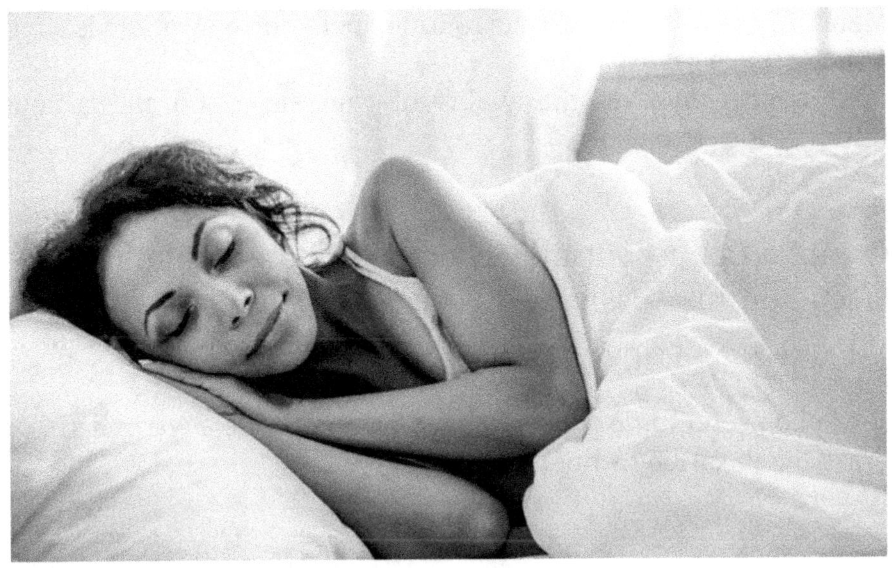

Explore the healing power of sleep on this journey, where the night becomes a refuge for repair and rebirth. Let the wisdom of rest guide you toward a future where each night's embrace supports a life of enduring vitality and health as we navigate the landscape of sleep and recovery.

Recuperation and sleep are vital for healthy aging. Sleep habits might change as people age, and the body's ability to recover from daily activities may deteriorate.

The following tips can help you age gracefully by encouraging improved sleep and recovery:

Maintain a regular sleep routine.
Maintain a regular sleep-wake routine, including on weekends.

Consistency improves the quality of your sleep and allows your internal clock to balance.

Create a Calm Bedtime Schedule: Create a calming pre-sleep routine to signal to your body that it is time to relax.

It can be useful to do things like read a book, take a warm bath, or practice relaxation techniques.

Enhance your sleeping environment.
1. Make your bedroom silent, dark, and cold.
2. Purchase a supportive mattress and pillows to ensure a pleasant night's sleep.

Limit your screen time before bedtime.

Limit your time on computers, phones, and tablets to at least an hour before bedtime.
Blue light generated by screens can disrupt the production of melatonin, the sleep hormone.

Keep Moving During the Day:

Exercise regularly, but avoid vigorous activity shortly before bedtime.
Regular exercise can improve your overall health and sleep quality.

Consciously Consuming Food:

Pay attention to your eating habits, especially at night. Avoid heavy meals right before bed.
Excessive consumption of alcohol and caffeine may disrupt sleep patterns.

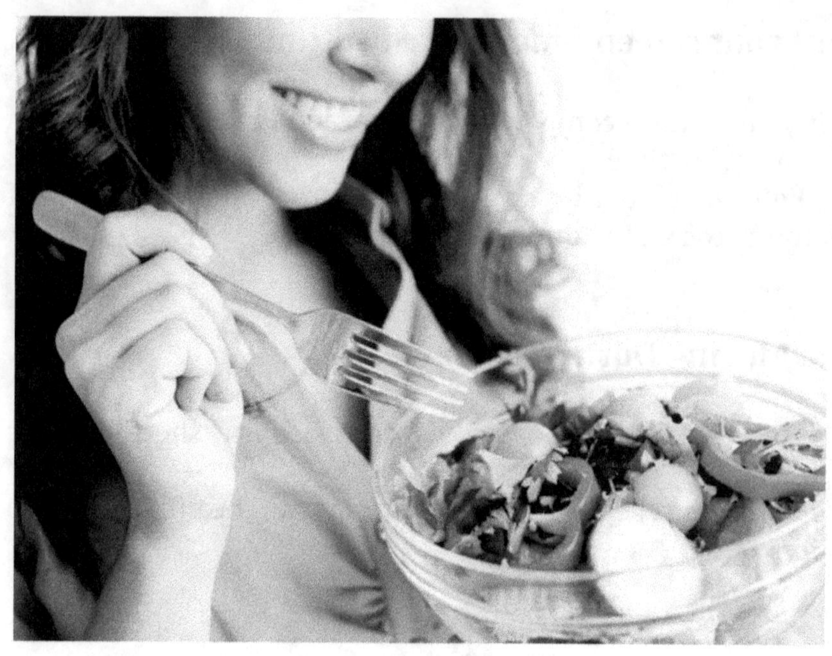

Maintain hydration.

Keep yourself hydrated during the day, but try to limit your fluid intake close to bedtime to reduce the likelihood of waking up needing to use the restroom.

Control your stress.

Use stress-reduction techniques like yoga, deep breathing, and meditation.
Prolonged stress might impair one's capacity to sleep and overall health.

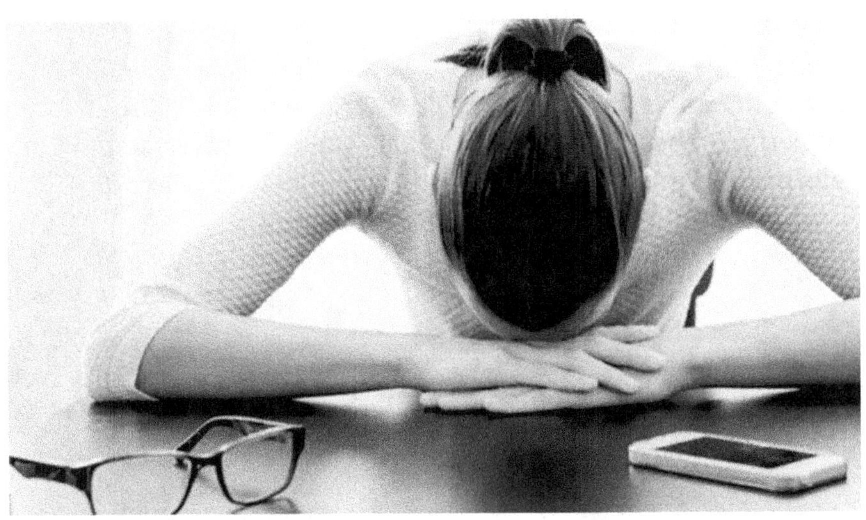

Think of napping.

In a short period of time (20–30 minutes), you can obtain a quick energy boost without losing your evening sleep.

Avoid extended naps and naps straight before bedtime.

Make recuperation a primary priority.

Allow your body adequate time to recover after physical activity.

To avoid overexertion, add rest days to your training schedule and listen to your body's cues.

Relationship to Others:

Maintain contact with friends and perform activities that make you happy.

Strong social bonds can boost mental wellness, leading to better sleep.

Frequent examinations:

Consult a healthcare practitioner regularly to address any underlying health conditions that may be interfering with sleep or recovery.

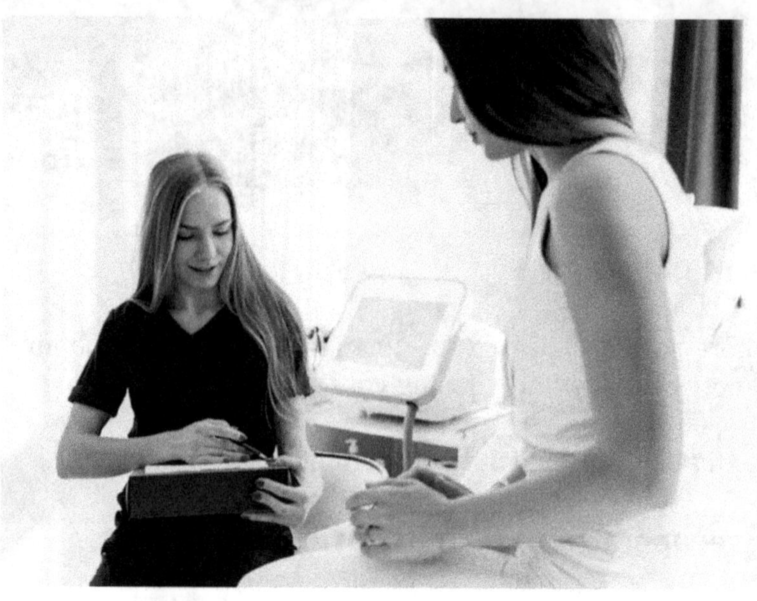

Remember that everyone's demands are different, so listen to your body and alter these suggestions to fit your scenario. If your sleep problems persist, you should consult a doctor.

Chapter 6: Stress Management for Healthy Aging

Stress appears as a silent but powerful orchestrator in the complicated dance of healthy aging, changing the cadence of our well-being. Chapter 6 deconstructs the rich tapestry of stress, investigating its impact on aging, providing stress-reduction practices based on mindfulness and relaxation, and directing you toward the development of a balanced and stress-resilient lifestyle.

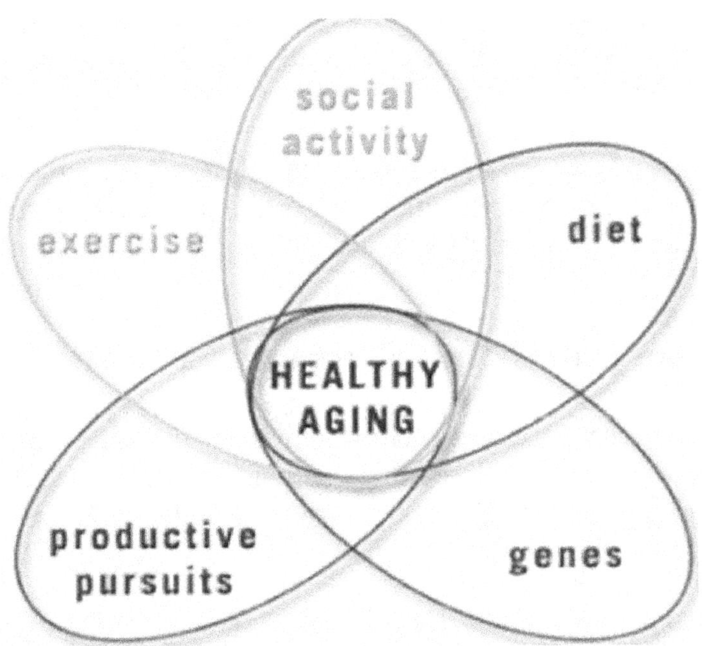

1. Recognizing the Effects of Stress on Aging

Stress, an ever-present companion on life's journey, has a significant impact on the aging process. This section dives into the complex relationship between stress and aging, examining how chronic stress can hasten the wear and tear on the body and mind. Understanding the varied impact of stress becomes a critical step in building a life of enduring vitality, from its influence on cellular aging to its consequences for general health.

2. Stress-reduction strategies, such as Mindfulness and Relaxation Exercises

Armed with knowledge about the effects of stress, we enter the arena of stress reduction, where mindfulness and relaxation techniques appear as effective tools. This chapter presents practical ways to soothe the nervous system, calm the mind, and relieve stress.

These practices, which range from mindful breathing exercises to progressive muscular relaxation, act as a compass, directing you towards a state of calm and resilience in the face of life's obstacles.

3. Developing a Stress-Resilient and Balanced Lifestyle

Beyond individual stress-reduction activities, the art of cultivating a lifestyle that promotes balance and resilience exists. This section delves into the components of a stress-resilient lifestyle, including nutrition, exercise, and social interactions.

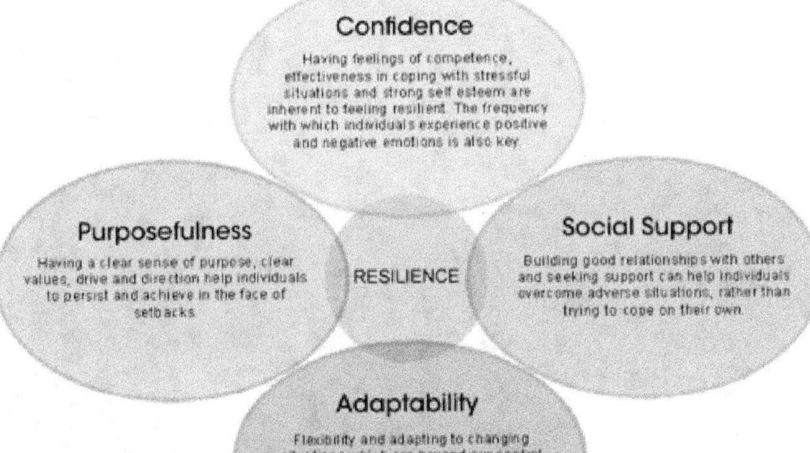

By connecting everyday behaviors with stress-reduction concepts, you embark on a journey to construct a life that not only withstands but also flourishes in the face of time's challenges. This all-encompassing approach to stress management becomes a cornerstone of good aging.

Remember that the path to resilience is an ongoing journey as we negotiate the landscape of stress and its role in aging. You may create a life that elegantly weathers the storms of stress by understanding, practicing, and making deliberate decisions, allowing you to relish each moment with a heart and mind free of unneeded tension. Join us as we delve into the art of stress management for healthy aging—a talent that serves as both a shield against the rigors of time and a key to unlocking a life of enduring well-being.

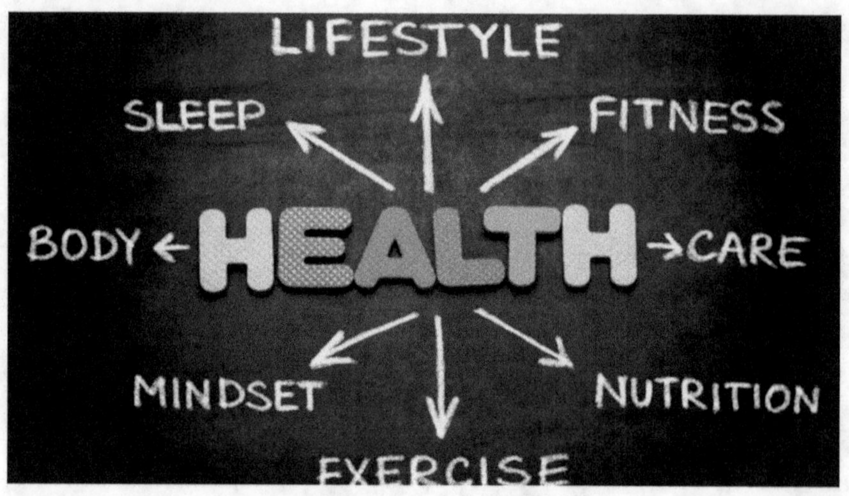

Since chronic stress can have a detrimental effect on one's physical and mental health, effective stress management is essential for healthy aging.

The following advice will help you cope with stress as you get older:

Frequent Exercise

Meditation and mindfulness:

Progressive muscle relaxation and deep breathing techniques can also aid in fostering mental calm.

Maintain social networks:
Increase the number of trustworthy friends, neighbors, and family members in your life.

Social support enhances emotional health and functions as a potent stress reducer.

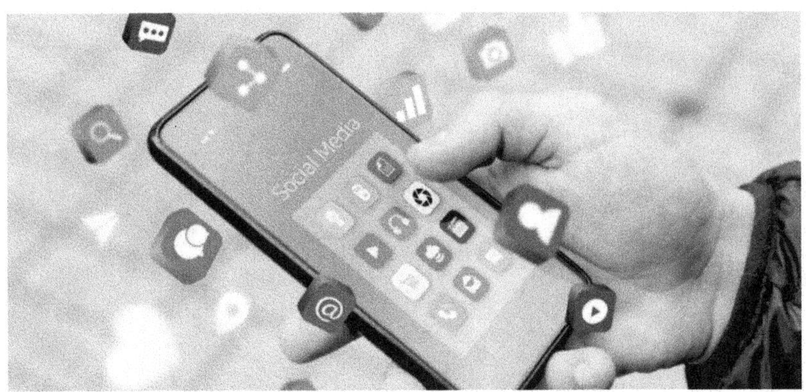

Establish reasonable objectives.

Set priorities for your work and divide it into doable chunks.
Set priorities for your job to prevent feeling overburdened.

Effective time management:

Set priorities and organize your tasks to help you manage your time better.
Recognize when to say no and delegate responsibility to others.

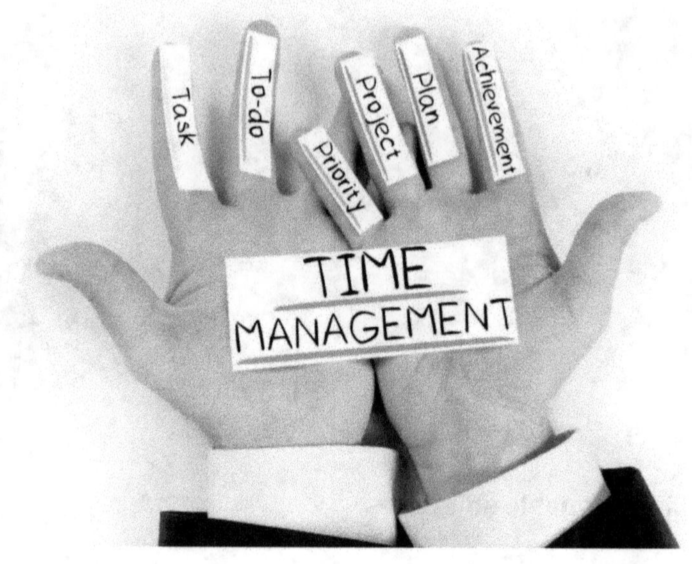

Good Living Practices:

A balanced diet rich in fruits, vegetables, and whole grains is what you should aim for.
Overindulgence in caffeine and alcohol can cause tension and interfere with sleep.

Sufficient Sleep:

Make sure you get enough pleasant sleep every night.
Create a calming evening ritual to encourage sound sleep.

Laugh and enjoy yourself.

Play games that make you laugh and feel happy.
Laughter eases stress and causes endorphins to be released.

Understand how to control your expectations.

Recognize that circumstances beyond your control may emerge from time to time.
Find appropriate coping mechanisms for uncertainty and concentrate on the things you can control.

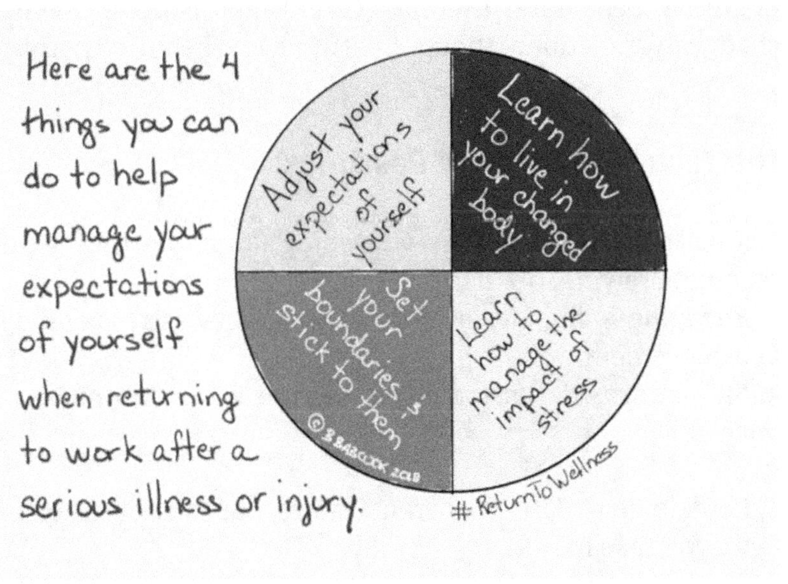

Body-Mind Techniques:

Investigate movement and concentration techniques such as tai chi or qigong.
These techniques help lessen stress and enhance general well-being.

Therapy based on cognitive behavior (CBT):

Consider going to counseling or therapy if you're finding it tough to
manage long-term stress.

Cognitive behavioral therapy (CBT) helps patients identify and change dysfunctional thought patterns and behavior patterns.

Interests and Inactive Pastimes:

1. Take part in the things you enjoy doing, be they gardening, reading, drawing, or anything else.
2. Engaging in hobbies offers a way to relieve stress and a feeling of achievement.
3. Stay informed, but try not to read or watch too much news at once.

4. Remain up to date on current affairs, but restrict the quantity of news you take in.
5. Restrict your exposure to upsetting news, especially right before bed.

Expert Assistance:

● If stress becomes intolerable, consult a mental health specialist.

● Counselors and therapists can offer coping mechanisms in addition to emotional support.

It's critical to understand that stress management is a personal process and that various stress-reduction techniques are effective for various people. To determine which strategy works best for you, try a few alternative ways. Do not hesitate to seek professional assistance if stress continues or becomes intolerable.

Chapter 7: Social Connections and Emotional Well-Being

In the complicated tapestry of healthy aging, the threads of social ties and emotional well-being weave together to generate a bright mosaic of resilience and fulfillment. Chapter 7 unravels the fundamental impact of social interactions on healthy aging, uncovers ways for preserving and establishing meaningful connections, and discusses the intricacies of emotional well-being and mental health among the aging population.

1. Exploring the Role of Social Relationships in Healthy Aging

Social relationships stand as pillars of strength, influencing the quality of life and general well-being as individuals age. This section looks into the inherent significance of social relationships in healthy aging, studying how companionship, community, and a sense of belonging contribute to mental and emotional resilience.

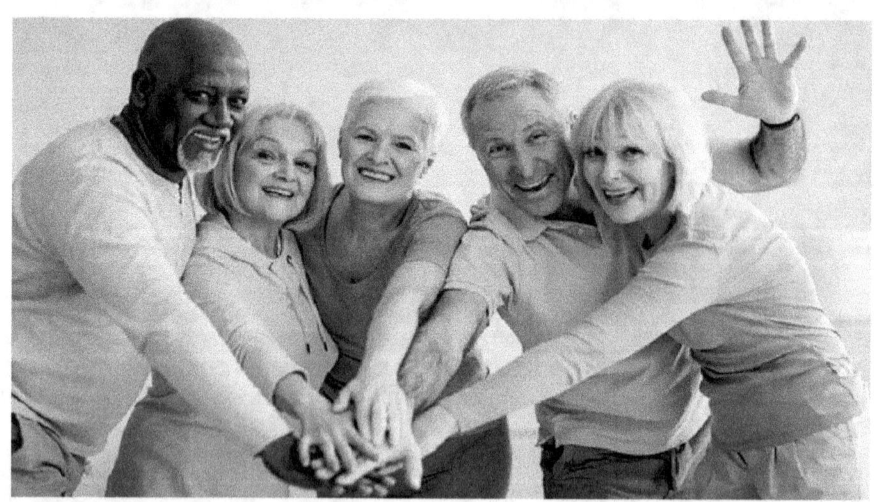

We reveal the science behind social interactions, illuminating their impact on cognitive function, stress reduction, and general life happiness. Through this exploration, you will come to understand the crucial role that social relationships play in the path of good aging.

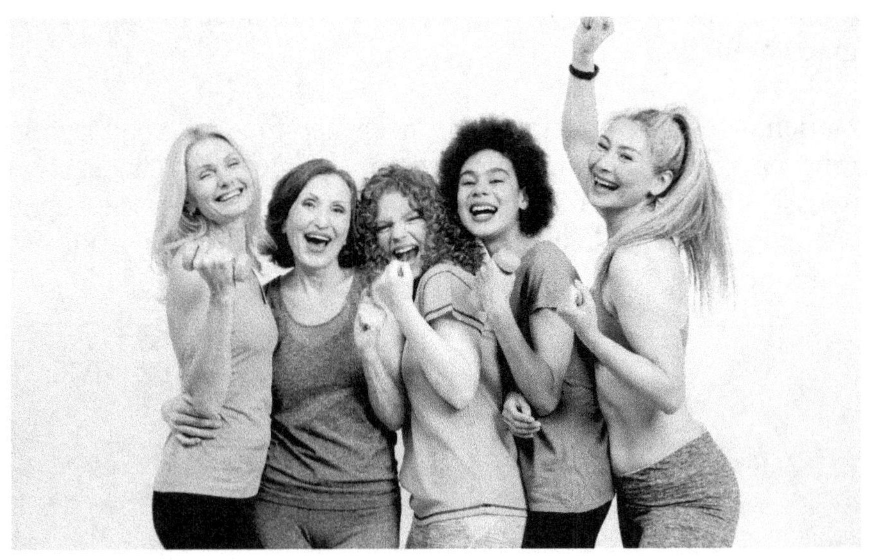

2. Strategies for Maintaining and Fostering Social Connections

Nurturing and sustaining social ties is an art that requires intentionality and commitment. This chapter presents practical ways for preserving and fostering meaningful connections as the years unfold. From community participation to harnessing technology for connection, these techniques serve as a roadmap to weave the threads of social relationships into the fabric of your daily life.

By embracing these activities, you set the way for a future rich in companionship, shared experiences, and emotional support—a future where the tapestry of social connections becomes an enduring source of strength.

3. Addressing Emotional Well-Being and Mental Health in the Aging Population

Emotional well-being stands as a cornerstone of good aging, influencing mental health and general life pleasure. This section discusses the distinct emotional landscapes within the aging population, offering insights into the problems and opportunities for emotional well-being.

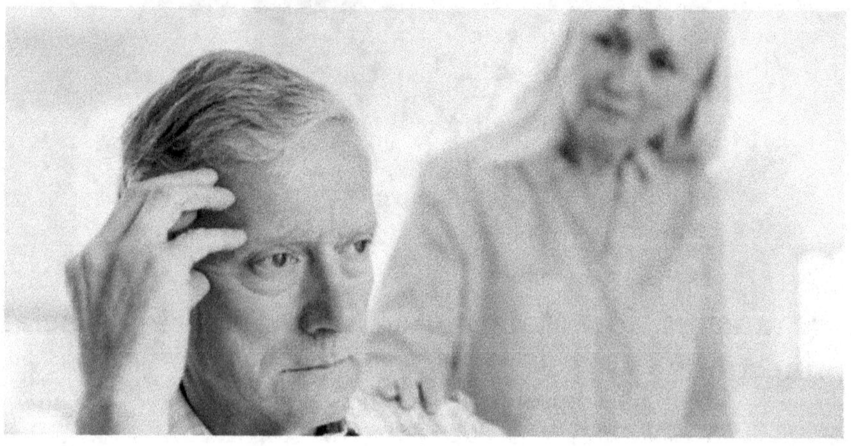

From coping with life transitions to building a positive mentality, we explore techniques that foster emotional resilience and enhance mental health. By embracing emotional well-being as an intrinsic element of healthy aging, you unlock the possibility for a meaningful and emotionally rich later life.

As we travel the worlds of social connections and emotional well-being, remember that the journey is not lonesome. The ties you form and the emotional landscapes you navigate contribute to the mosaic of a life well lived. Join us in this examination of the heart and soul, where social ties and emotional well-being become the brushstrokes that paint a portrait of enduring vitality and fulfillment in the fabric of healthy aging.

Maintaining social relationships is critical for emotional well-being and overall health, especially as we age. Here are some strategies for fostering social ties and improving emotional well-being as we age:

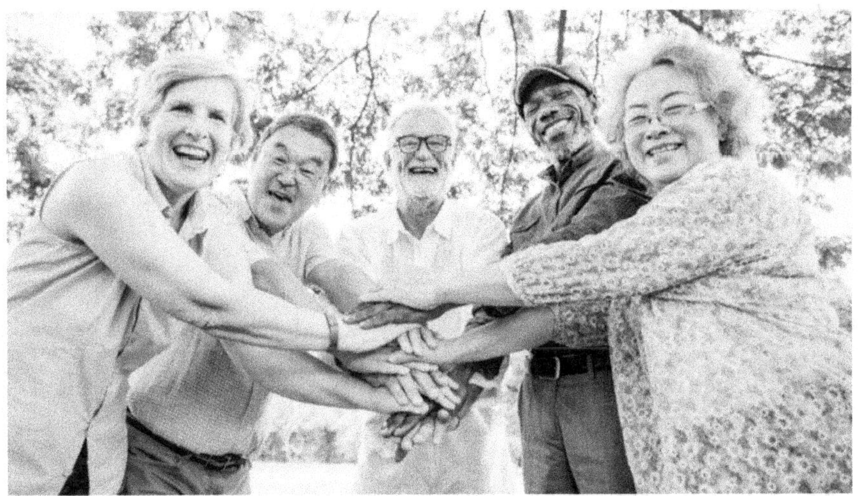

Maintain contact with friends and family.

● Regularly communicate with family members and friends, whether in person, over the phone, or through video calls.

● Plan frequent visits or outings to strengthen ties.

● Participate in social groups.

● Participate in clubs, community groups, or organizations that match your interests.

This offers the chance to network with new people who have similar interests and passions.

Offer assistance:

● Volunteering can help foster a good self-image and a sense of purpose.

● It also enables you to establish connections with people who are dedicated to the same cause.

● Participate in social events.

● Attend community events, social gatherings, and cultural activities.

These gatherings provide chances to socialize and have deep conversations with new individuals.

Accept Technology:

● Stay in touch with loved ones through technology, particularly if distance is an issue.

● Video calls, social media, and messaging apps can help to close the distance and preserve ties.

Develop new connections.

● Be willing to meet new people, no matter your age.

● Join seminars or workshops to pick up new skills and network with like-minded individuals.

● Continue to participate in the community.

● Participate in local events, attend neighborhood meetings, and engage in community activities.

This can improve links within the community and foster a sense of belonging.

Give Your Wisdom a Share:

It can be beneficial for both sides to mentor someone or take part in intergenerational activities.

Use creativity to express yourself.

Connecting with people who have similar interests and finding a powerful emotional outlet can both be achieved through creative expression.

Participate in support groups.

Become a member of support groups focused on particular life stages, medical issues, or hobbies.
These communities offer a forum for experience sharing and emotional support.

Engage in Active Listening:

Engage in active listening when interacting with people to get insight into their viewpoints and experiences.
Having effective listening skills improves relationships with others.

Seek expert assistance.

If you continue to feel lonely or isolated, go to a mental health professional.
Therapists can provide assistance and solutions to increase emotional well-being.

Honor significant anniversaries:

Celebrate significant life events, accomplishments, and turning points with loved ones.
Social ties are strengthened by sharing these events.

Encourage good connections.

Keep yourself surrounded by positive and encouraging individuals.

Develop a network of relationships that enhance your emotional health.

Keep in mind that the caliber of your social networks frequently matters more than their quantity. Building and maintaining meaningful relationships can greatly contribute to emotional well-being and provide a support system as people age.

Chapter 8: Preventive Health Measures

Prevention emerges as a powerful brushstroke in the mosaic of healthy aging, maintaining the canvas of well-being and energy. Chapter 8 unveils a study of preventative health measures for older persons, including an overview of critical health exams and vaccines. We delve into the necessity of frequent health check-ups, stressing early diagnosis of age-related health concerns. Additionally, this chapter gives practical ideas for proactive health management and disease prevention, helping you to negotiate the path of aging with foresight and resilience.

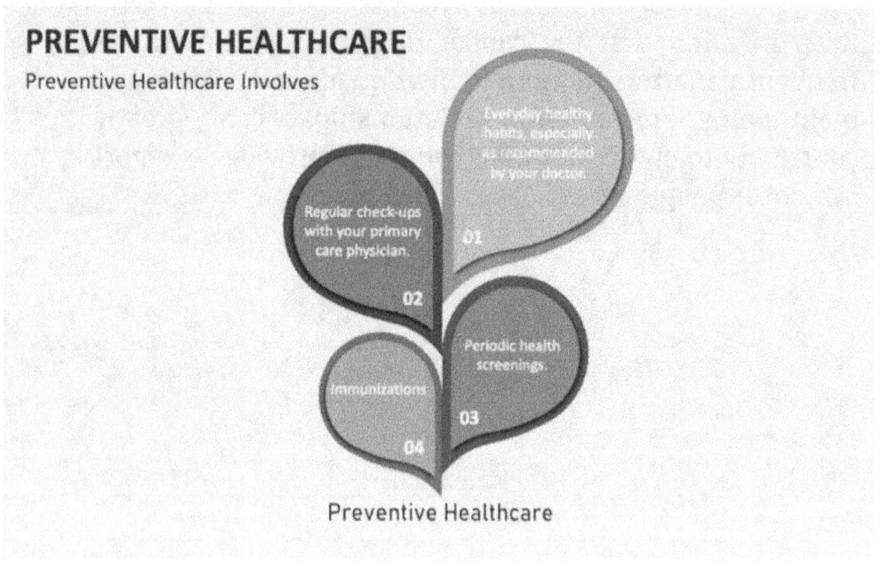

Preventive Healthcare

1. Overview of Preventive Health Screenings and Vaccinations for Older Adults

Prevention begins with information, and this part provides a complete overview of the preventative health strategies designed for older people.

We review crucial health screenings that play a pivotal role in the early detection of probable health disorders. Additionally, the relevance of immunizations in defending against infectious diseases is revealed, building a foundation for proactive health care. By knowing and prioritizing these preventive steps, you lay the framework for a health-focused path as you age.

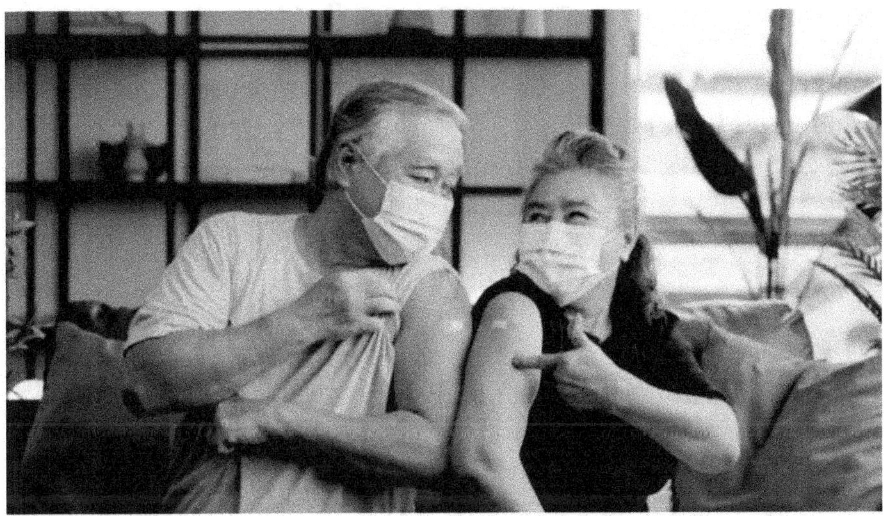

2. The importance of regular health check-ups and early detection of age-related health issues

Regular health check-ups act as compass points, directing you down the path of well-being. This chapter underlines the significance of routine health checkups, stressing their role in the early diagnosis of age-related health concerns. From blood pressure monitoring to cholesterol screenings, we unravel the major components of health check-ups targeted at older people. By implementing regular health assessments into your wellness regimen, you become an active participant in your health journey, equipped with the knowledge to address possible concerns before they escalate.

3. Tips for Proactive Health Management and Disease Prevention

Proactive health management is a cornerstone of aging with vitality. This section gives practical ideas for assuming a proactive posture in illness prevention. From adopting a healthy lifestyle to understanding genetic predispositions, these tactics enable you to take care of your health. By fostering habits that support well-being and resilience, you create a framework for a future marked by proactive health management and a lower risk of age-related disorders.

Remember that every proactive decision we make now is a step toward long-term, sustainable well-being down the road as we continue our investigation into preventative health practices. Join us in unraveling the layers of prevention, where information becomes a shield and proactive decisions become the guiding lights on the journey of good aging.

Here are some other preventive health interventions specifically designed to promote good aging:

Bone Health:

Calcium and vitamin D should be consumed in sufficient amounts to promote healthy bones.

Weight-bearing workouts and resistance training can help you maintain your bone density and strength.

Vision and hearing tests:

Regular eye and hearing exams are recommended to detect age-related changes in vision and hearing.

Correct any faults with corrective devices such as glasses or hearing aids.

Immunizations:

Keep up with recommended vaccinations, including those designed specifically for older people, such as flu and pneumonia vaccines.

Immunizations can assist in avoiding some diseases and their consequences.

Cardiovascular Health:

Adopt heart-healthy habits such as eating a balanced diet, exercising regularly, and staying at a healthy weight.

Monitor and manage blood pressure and cholesterol levels to lower your risk of cardiovascular disease.

Cognitive health:

Do things that will keep your mind active to help your brain work better.
Stay socially active, explore hobbies, and stretch your brain by learning new skills.

Balanced Diet:

A nutrient-dense, well-balanced diet should include fruits, vegetables, whole grains, lean proteins, and healthy fats.

Pay attention to portion sizes and age-specific nutritional standards.

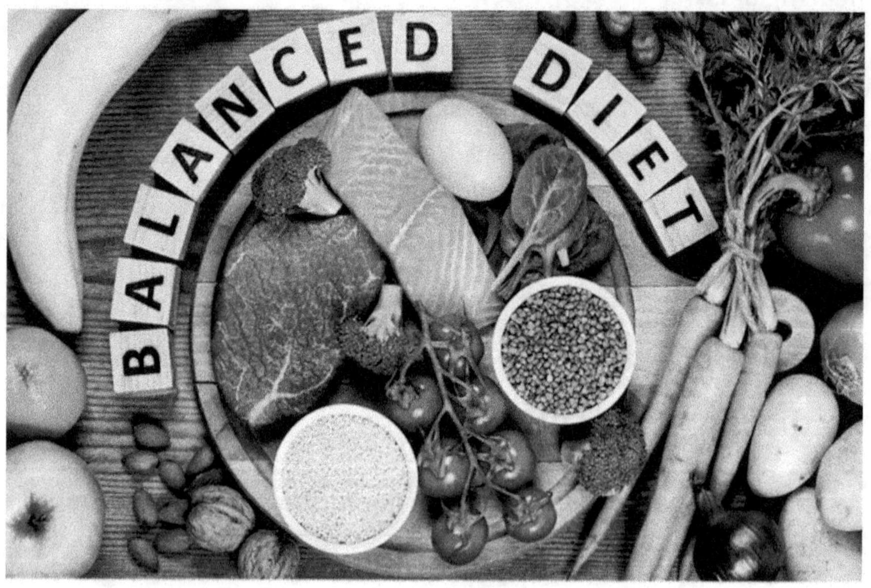

Hydration:
Stay hydrated, as dehydration can lead to a variety of health complications.

Be mindful of your water consumption, especially in warmer regions or during vigorous exertion.

Regular physical activity:

Cardio, strength training, and stretching should all be part of your workout routine.

Regular physical activity helps to preserve muscle mass, joint flexibility, and general mobility.

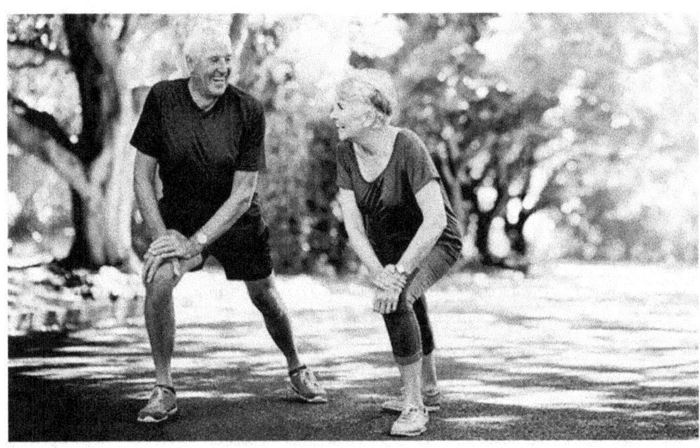

Sleep hygiene:

Prioritize proper sleep hygiene by sticking to a consistent sleep schedule and creating a pleasant sleeping environment. Address any sleep-related concerns, such as insomnia or sleep apnea, with the help of a healthcare provider.

Prevent falls:

Make use of handrails, keep your living area clutter-free, and engage in activities that improve your balance to prevent falls.

Regular exercise helps improve balance and lower the chance of falling.

Screening for cancer and chronic illnesses:

Follow the prescribed cancer tests and wellness checks, such as mammograms, colonoscopies, and screenings for diabetes.

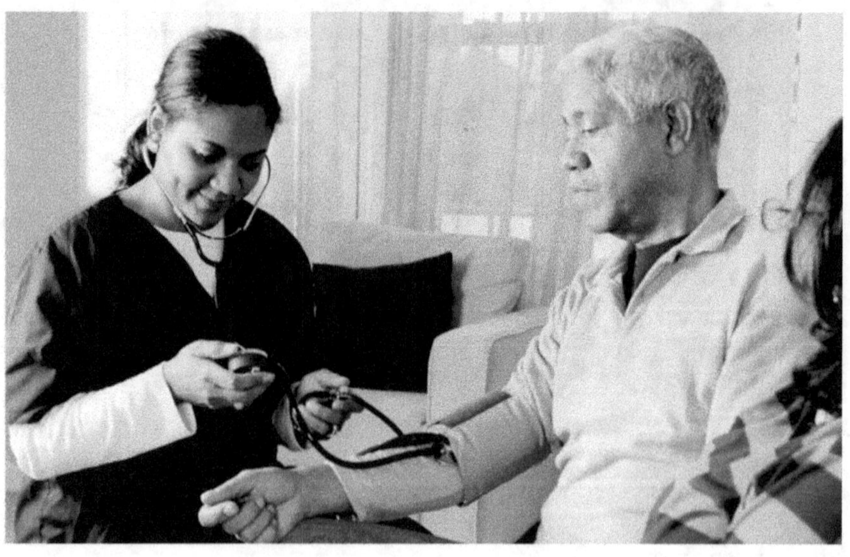

Mindfulness and Stress Management:

Practice mindfulness, meditation, and relaxation practices to improve your stress management.

Chronic stress can have an impact on both physical and mental health; therefore, good coping skills are crucial.

Social Connections:

Stay socially connected to avoid feelings of solitude.

Maintain close relationships with friends and family, and aggressively seek out opportunities for social interaction.

Maintain mental health:

Make mental health a priority by getting help when you need it and taking care of mental health issues like anxiety and sadness.

Regular mental health check-ins with healthcare practitioners can help.

Remember that all recommendations should be adapted to your own health needs and concerns. Consult a healthcare expert for individualized advice based on your medical history and current situation. A healthy approach to age takes into account the well-being of your body, mind, and social life.

Chapter 9: Adapting to Lifestyle Changes

Adaptation is a crucial element in the tapestry of good aging, as it helps navigate the changes and adjustments that come with being older. Chapter 9 is a guide to embracing change, discussing the importance of adapting to evolving situations and abilities. It unfolds strategies for maintaining independence and preserving the quality of life while also shedding light on the resources and support systems available for aging people and their families.

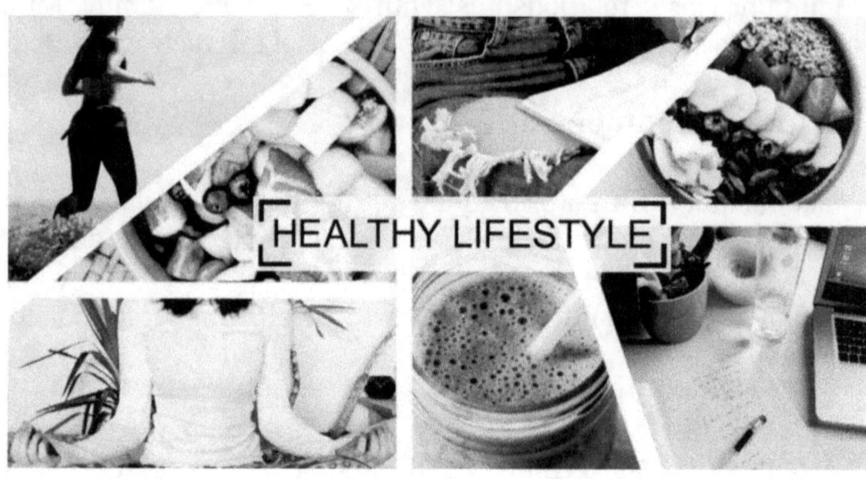

1. Discussing the Importance of Adapting to Changing Circumstances and Abilities

As the hands of time continue their gentle march, the landscape of life shifts and changes. This part explores the value of acknowledging and adapting to these transformations. From physical abilities to lifestyle situations, adapting becomes a cornerstone in the journey of healthy aging. We delve into the wisdom of embracing change, noting that adaptation is not a surrender but a dynamic response to the ebb and flow of life. By knowing the significance of adaptation, you pave the way for a resilient and fulfilling later life.

2. Strategies for Maintaining Independence and Quality of Life

Independence and quality of life are the jewels that adorn the crown of a healthy age. This chapter unfolds a spectrum of strategies meant to maintain independence and uphold a high quality of life. From incorporating assistive technologies to creating a supportive living environment, these strategies empower you to manage the changing landscape with grace and autonomy. By implementing these methods, you cultivate a lifestyle that honors both your capabilities and aspirations, ensuring that each day is a celebration of independence and well-being.

3. Resources and Support Systems for Aging Individuals and Their Families

No journey is made alone, and in the chapter on healthy aging, support systems and resources become invaluable companions. This section illuminates the wealth of resources available for aging people and their families. From neighborhood organizations to healthcare services, we explore avenues that provide guidance, assistance, and a sense of belonging.
By tapping into these resources, you build a robust network that fortifies you and your loved ones on the

path of healthy aging, building a collective strength that enhances the quality of life.

Here are some suggestions for adjusting to lifestyle modifications for healthy aging:

Embrace a positive mindset.

Approach aging positively and consider it a normal part of life.

Concentrate on the opportunities and experiences associated with each period of life.

Stay active and exercise regularly.

Adjust your workout regimen to reflect your current fitness level and any physical constraints.

To keep your strength, flexibility, and heart-healthy, try low-impact activities like walks, swimming, or tai chi.

Healthy food habits:

Adjust your diet to match shifting nutritional requirements. Consume a well-balanced diet focusing on nutrient-dense foods, and consult a nutritionist for individualized guidance.

Prioritize Sleep:

To encourage higher-quality sleep, modify your nightly schedule. Set a consistent bedtime, create a comfortable sleep environment, and discuss any sleep-related concerns with your healthcare physician.

Social Engagement:

Adapt to changes in social groups by actively seeking new friendships and maintaining existing relationships.

Take part in social activities and community events to stay connected.

Financial Planning:

Adjust your financial strategy to account for retirement and anticipated medical expenses.

Seek financial counsel to guarantee a pleasant and secure financial future.

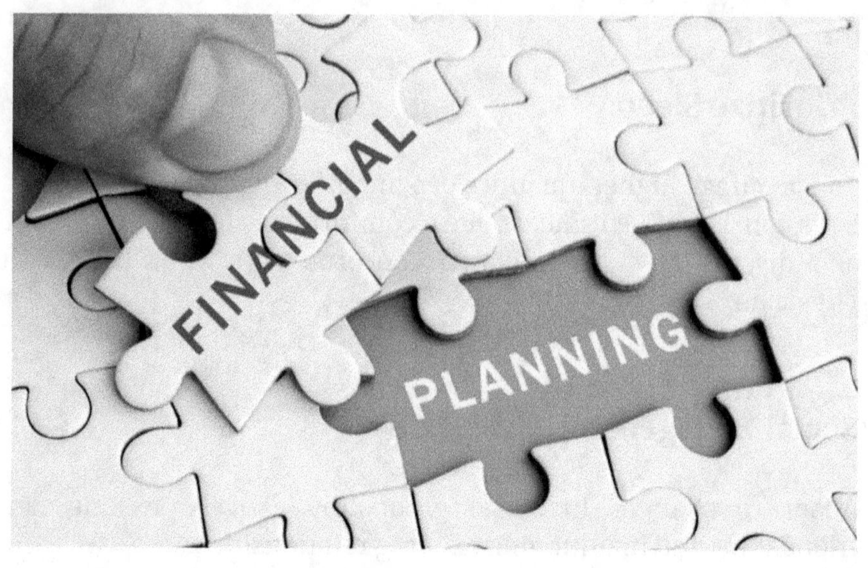

Regular health check-ups:

Adapt to changing health needs by booking regular check-ups and screenings.

Be open and honest with your healthcare providers about any changes or concerns you may have regarding your health.

Mindfulness and stress reduction:

Incorporate mindfulness and stress-reduction techniques into your daily life.

Mindfulness, meditation, and relaxation techniques can help enhance mental health.

Adapt your living environment.

Make changes to your home to increase safety and accessibility.

Consider railings, ramps, and adequate illumination to help prevent accidents.

Cognitive health:

Puzzles, games, and learning new abilities are all examples of mentally stimulating hobbies.
Maintain mental activity to enhance cognitive function and lower the risk of cognitive decline.

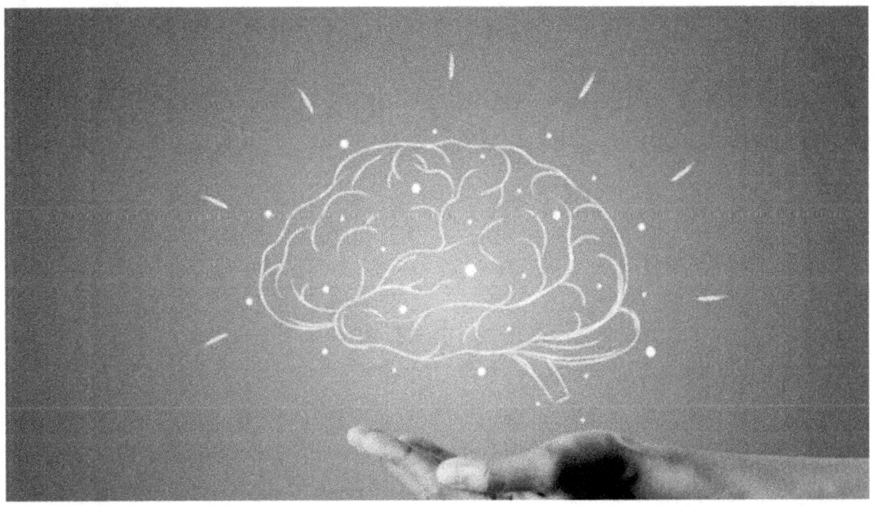

Tech-savvy adaptations:
Embrace technology to keep connected with loved ones, get health information, and engage in online activities.

Learn how to utilize cell phones, tablets, and computers to communicate and acquire information.

Pace yourself:

You should modify your daily routine to include relaxation and breaks.
Pace yourself to save energy and avoid burnout.

Accept and manage changes.

Accept that physical and mental changes are a normal aspect of aging.
Manage chronic diseases with the help of a healthcare expert and adjust your lifestyle accordingly.

Seek Support:

When you need emotional support and help, don't hesitate to reach out to friends, family, or support groups.
Recognize the value of a support system in adjusting to lifestyle changes.

Continue to learn and grow.

Develop a mentality of constant learning and personal improvement.

Discover new interests, take classes, and remain curious about the world around you.

Flexibility, resiliency, and a proactive approach to well-being are necessary for adjusting to changes in lifestyle. By making conscious modifications and seeking support when needed, individuals can age gracefully and retain a satisfying and healthy existence.

As we navigate the terrain of lifestyle changes, remember that adaptation is not a solitary endeavor—it's a symphony of adjustments, backed by the rich harmony of resources and relationships. Join us in this study of adaptation, where change becomes an opportunity and the journey of healthy aging transforms into a masterpiece of resilience, independence, and enduring well-being.

Conclusion

In the final chapter of "Healthy Aging: Strategies for Maintaining Health and Fitness as You Age," we arrive at a point where the threads of wisdom, guidance, and inspiration come together to weave a tapestry of enduring well-being. Let us review the essential healthy aging methods mentioned in this transforming journey, encourage a proactive and positive approach to aging, and emphasize the importance of a holistic lifestyle as the foundation for sustaining health and fitness in later years.

1. Key Strategies for a Healthy Aging Synthesis

We've discovered a treasure trove of tactics meticulously created to improve the aging process. Each chapter has provided insights, practical recommendations, and empowering knowledge, ranging from comprehending the physiological changes in the aging process to embracing preventive health practices. Nutrition, exercise, mental well-being, sleep, stress management, social connections, and preventative health measures are all part of this holistic pathway. Consider these tactics as stepping stones leading you to a future filled with vitality, resilience, and fulfillment.

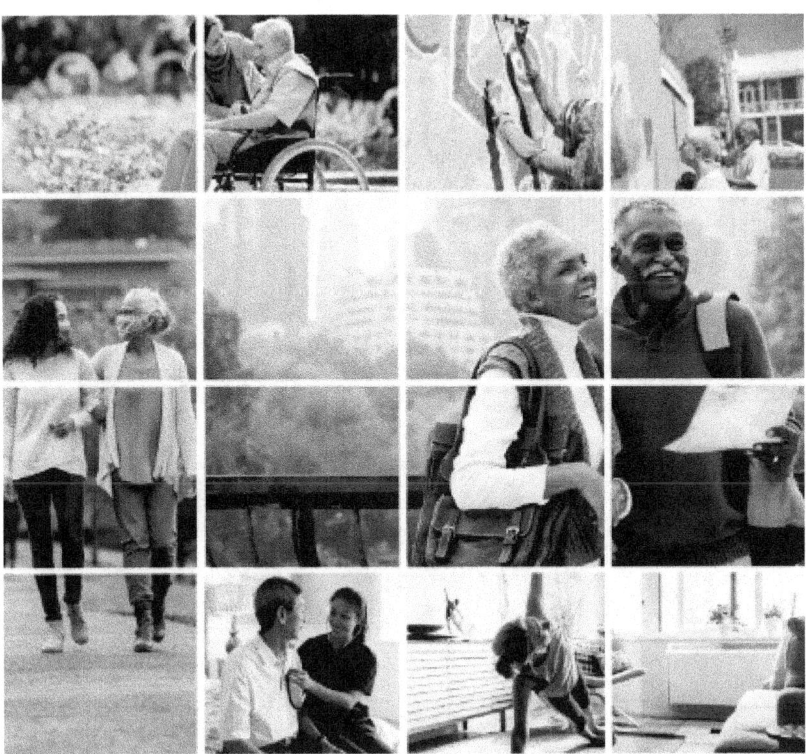

2. Promoting a Proactive and Positive Aging Approach

Growing older is a dynamic journey that changes with each passing day, rather than a destination. Let us take a proactive and constructive approach to aging in this final chapter. Change your focus from a yearly count to an appreciation for the rich tapestry of experiences, wisdom, and progress that each year delivers. Positive thinking acts as a lighthouse, illuminating the route forward and transforming each day into an opportunity for self-discovery and delight. Accept the voyage with open arms, and rejoice in the blessings that come with the passing of time.

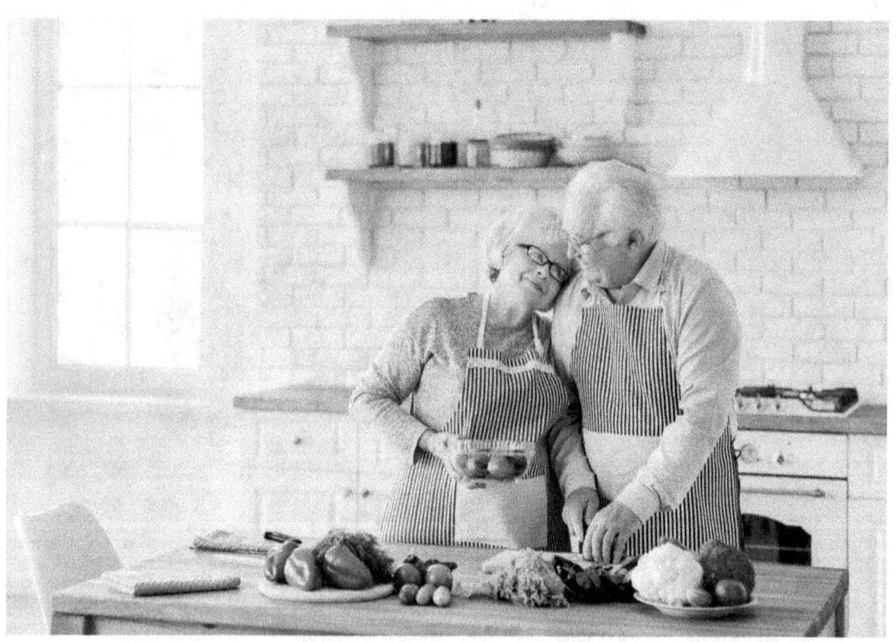

3. Emphasizing the Value of a Holistic Lifestyle

As we say goodbye to these pages, the overriding message is one of holistic living—a way of life that balances the body, mind, and spirit. The interdependence of nutrition, exercise, mental health, and social ties creates the foundation of long-term health and fitness.

Reinforce your commitment to a lifestyle that looks beyond individual components, acknowledging the synergy that occurs when all aspects of well-being are cultivated. The holistic approach captures the essence of good aging by ensuring that all aspects of your life contribute to robust and meaningful later life.

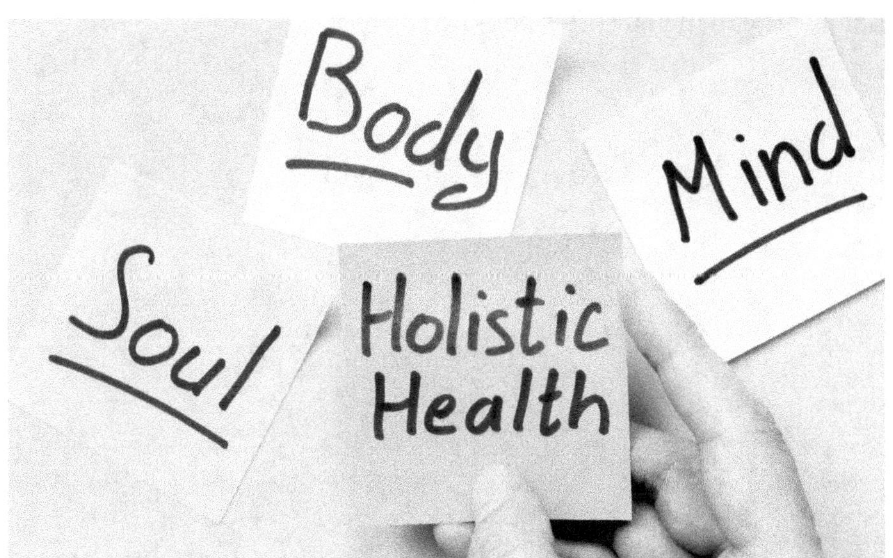

Finally, "Healthy Aging" is more than simply a book; it is a companion on your journey to a future full of health, energy, and purpose. May you discover inspiration, direction, and empowerment inside these pages as they form a part of your personal narrative. Allow the ideas outlined to act as tools in your toolbox, assisting you in creating a life in which each passing year is a witness to the beauty of aging gracefully and thriving in later years.

Here's to a bright future full of health, happiness, and the unyielding spirit of healthy aging. Cheers to the exciting pages that await you in your life's book!

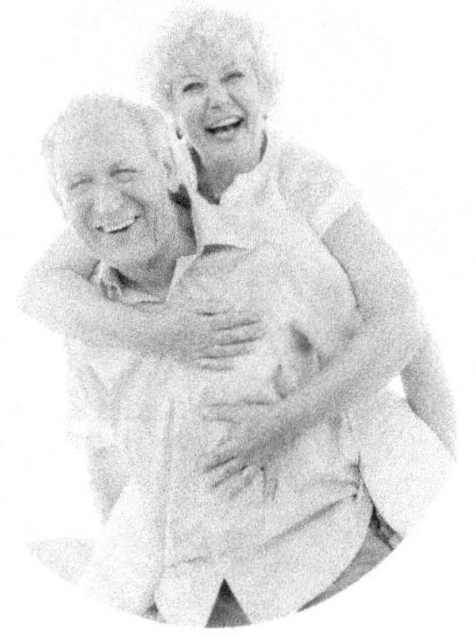

Aging Healthy for better living